49

MORECAMBE BAY HOSPITALS NHS TRUST

ONE IN THREE

One in Three

A SON'S JOURNEY
INTO THE
HISTORY AND SCIENCE
OF CANCER

Adam Wishart

PROFILE BOOKS

First published in Great Britain in 2006 by
PROFILE BOOKS LTD
3A Exmouth House
Pine Street
Exmouth Market
London ECIR OJH
www.profilebooks.com

Extract from 'Miss Gee' from *Collected Poems* by W. H. Auden (p. 73)
printed here with kind permission of Faber and Faber.
Extract from 'How to behave with the ill' reproduced with the kind permission of
Julia Darling's family. The poem is published in *The Poetry Cure*, by Julia Darling and
Cynthia Fuller (eds) (Newcastle University/Bloodaxe Books, 2005).

1 3 5 7 9 10 8 6 4 2

Printed and bound in Great Britain by
Clays, Bungay, Suffolk

The moral right of the author has been asserted.

A CIP catalogue record for this book is available from the British Library.

ISBN-10 1 86197 752 2
ISBN-13 978 1 86197 752 6

The text in this book is set in Baskerville – one of Dad's favourite types. I think he liked
the idea that the type was designed in Birmingham, the city that became his home. The
headings are in Albertus, one of the first faces that Dad bought when he began printing
as a hobby in the 1970s. When Dad began to teach me to print, one of the lessons was
setting our names in it.

The ONE IN THREE on the front of the jacket is from a font of unspecified sans serif
wood-letter which Dad bought in the early 1980s. I printed the title badly, with too
much ink, on his old Albion press, in November 2005.

For Dad

Contents

Introduction

I CLING TO MY DAD'S ENORMOUS HAND. With long strides, we are rushing through London. I am six. I am sometimes catching my step, sometimes just being lifted by his forward thrust. I am wearing a bright yellow cape, with a sailor's hat to keep the rain off, and at every puddle I splash the rushing Christmas shoppers. Dad scolds me, but I know he doesn't mean it: we are a tight pair. We are coming from an exhibition about some ancient civilisation at the Royal Academy, where he had lifted me high above the crowds so that I could see the twinkling gold swords. Now we have to get somewhere, probably the coffee-bean shop in Soho, for he has very particular tastes. Although we are in a hurry, as we round a corner he stops sharply and I charge straight into his camel-hair coat. It is warm and wet. We have paused because he wants to tell me a story of a man called John Snow whose name and picture is on a pub sign across the road.

Many years ago, Dad says, Dr Snow had hundreds of patients dying of a particularly vicious disease. As Snow had no idea what caused it, he could neither treat nor prevent it. So to discover what connected the patients, he drew a map of London and placed dots where each one lived. Dad sweeps his hand down Broadwick Street, explaining the map:

here was dark with dots, but further away the dots became sparser. Dad asks me what linked them. I scratch my head. The doctor didn't know either. So he questioned the families about their lives. With a flourish, Dad points to the spot where a water pump once stood, and says that Snow realised that all the ill people had used this pump. Some liked the taste of its water so much that they had even travelled from afar. To stop the disease, Snow simply removed the handle of the pump. Nobody became ill again.

Dad tells me it was the first piece of work on demonology. I ask him what kind of demons, but he only laughs.

It amused him that I had misheard the word 'epidemiology', the science of epidemics, especially since this was a subject he taught to his statistics students.

Being taught about the cholera epidemic of 1854 is my first memory of Dad's quest to educate me – even though in hindsight Dad's story was a rather mythologised and child-friendly version of history. From then on, he was always telling me stories about scientists, mathematicians and revolutionaries, from Marie Curie to Benjamin Franklin. From my adolescence it was our habit to stay up late and, with Mum in bed, to sit talking about these things at the kitchen table. For two men who never spoke about their feelings, our intimacy consisted in sharing our interests in politics, history or the progress of science. If I knew history, he thought, then I might be better able to navigate through my life because he had always used the past as a way to understand his place in the world.

For as long as I can remember, I was the one who would eventually leave the table. Dad would lock the doors and begin to turn off the lights. I would make my way to bed. The final part of the ritual was that he would open my door just enough for him to stick his head through and wish me goodnight. Then I would listen as he darkened the house before turning in.

Many years later, when Dad became ill, we began spending more time together again and we continued to tell those stories, although this time they would be about the scientists, doctors and patients who had struggled against cancer across the centuries. I searched for a book that we could both read and then discuss. There were memoirs of celebrities who had 'battled' through the disease, but I knew that Dad would have no interest in those. There were self-help guides that presented basic information but provided no wider context. There were books that described the science in detail, but they didn't seem to connect to the experience of being a patient. And there were academic histories, which did not seem to bring the past alive.

Even without a book to fall back on, Dad pondered the big questions. Why was there no cure yet, for instance? And I would search libraries for biographies of those who had tried and the reasons why they had failed. Dad would show me a newspaper cutting about the latest genetic cancer cures, and I would try to paint in the background with my recently acquired knowledge. It was like some game from my childhood, but with dark undertones, because the purpose was to provide a distraction from the blizzard of pain.

This book is, in part, the culmination of that journey. It tells the history of cancer medicine, from the Victorian surgical solution to the latest developments in gene therapy, through a dozen stories of scientific endeavour. These are stories of maverick doctors searching for a cure although their colleagues thought them to be charlatans, and of patients campaigning to stay alive. Running through them is a vein of the wider history of medicine, and of the development of science's understanding of human biology. At the same time, these stories address some of the basic questions that Dad and I had about cancer: what is the biology of the disease, how does a tumour grow, why is it so difficult to detect sometimes, and how does radiation or chemotherapy work?

Dad's illness mirrored these historical moments. At times, medicine's history had direct relevance to his own experience. At others, the spirit of some historical age seemed to resonate with the mood of the family. As a consequence, the story of Dad's illness forms a counterpoint to the broader history of humanity's struggle against cancer.

❧

It is almost four years since that moment when I was told that Dad was ill and I became filled with fear. I wish that I had known then what I know now. Because learning something about cancer calmed some of those terrors.

When I began writing this book, I thought not only that the disease was becoming more common, that more and more people were dying from it, but that medicine had failed to cure it. But as I met more doctors I realised that, in fact, the last decade has been historic for cancer research: death rates have been falling, in the UK, the US and across Europe, for the first time; and we now understand the biology of cancers in much greater detail than ever before. As a result, in the last few years the first treatments based on understanding the genetic mechanism of the disease have arrived on the market. Many doctors are therefore predicting that in just a few decades cancer will become a disease more like diabetes, one that we will live with rather than only die from.

Most importantly, this book has prepared me for the next time the disease strikes – whether that be within myself, against one of my friends or within a member of my family. I know that this will come, because one in three of us will develop the disease in our lifetimes. When we count our families, our friends and our work colleagues, it is evident that we will all be touched, in some way. And I have learnt that an amalgam of fear, archaic prejudices and ignorance is no way to deal with it. It is time that this disease is no longer shrouded by a dangerous taboo.

Adam Wishart
February 2006

Incipience:

the disease emerges

A s a child, I was haunted by the thought that Dad was about to die. Despite having the physique of an enormous bear – standing at six foot two, stoutly built, with a plume of wiry black hair – he was, I thought, fragile. Although when I was a child, he could lift me high above his head, it seemed even then as if he had been weakened by age and, like a ruined castle in the throes of collapse, as if he was in constant danger of toppling. Perhaps I had developed this impression because he was so much older than my friend's fathers. My anxiety reached its peak when I was eleven years old and he was to be away for three months on an academic sabbatical. In the days before his departure, I became convinced that he would die before I would see him again. The journey to the station, therefore, was to be my last time with him. So rather than chatting to him amiably, I began to trace his wrinkles and his eyes in the car's rear-view mirror. Like a diligent cartographer, I divided his face into sections and tried to memorise every contour and blemish in a desperate attempt to imprint his features on my mind. To this day, when I drive down that particular piece of road, flashes of his face pass through my thoughts.

By contrast, I felt no similar foreboding for my mother. There is nothing in her nature that hints at her mortality.

My worry about Dad did not recede as I grew older. When he stood waving goodbye to me outside our family home, when he wandered away into the crowds of a London street, or when his face disappeared into the distance as his train moved off, I often wondered if it would be the last time I would ever see him. One gesture, in particular, seemed to encapsulate the way I thought he would depart: as he walked away, hurrying to another appointment, he would thrust his hand into the air and, without looking back, wave goodbye. For years, each time he did that I presumed that it would be my last memory of him.

§♠.

Cancer has always existed among humans. When the first man stood upright on the plains of Africa more than a million years ago, he or one of his relations suffered from the disease: a fossilised jawbone that was excavated near Nairobi in 1932, for instance, contains the scar of what many believe to be a malignant tumour; the victim was either *Australopithecus* or *Homo erectus*, who both existed at the dawn of our species. The disease's filigrees have also left their marks on Egyptian mummies, on a 2,400-year-old Inca body, and on Bronze Age heads. One of the earliest written texts, a 110-page Egyptian scroll called the Ebers papyrus, from about 1600 BC, describes large, loathsome tumours of the leg. A thousand years later, Ayurvedic medical books from India reported mouth and throat tumours and described how to treat them. By 400 BC, Greek doctors had written about tumours of the breast, stomach, skin, cervix and rectum. For classification they used the word for crab, *carcinos* (hence *carcinoma*), apparently because of the way in which tumours – especially those of the breast – transform the skin into hard plates from which leg-like blood vessels protrude. In time, this word was Latinised to *cancer*.

Yet although cancer had been identified in ancient times, the disease was responsible for only a tiny proportion of all deaths: many more people were killed by smallpox, the plague and a variety of then unnamed infections. With an average lifespan of about thirty years, few would have lived long enough to develop a life-threatening tumour, whereas nowadays two-thirds of cancer cases occur in the over 65s. Even those cancers that were fatal usually went undiscovered because there were no tools to investigate inside the body's organs, and post-mortem examinations were eschewed because of beliefs and superstitions about the sanctity of the body. As such, cancer hardly touched the culture or the imaginations of the ancient world.

'Why these symptoms develop is not known by physicians themselves, let alone the masses,' wrote the celebrated physician of the Roman era, Galen, on the subject of cancer in AD 165; 'nor do physicians make systematic investigation; they simply announce what they think.' Galen was famous as the doctor to the Emperor Marcus Aurelius and for his public dissections of pigs (who would continue to scream until he theatrically cut their laryngeal nerve). But he was also a prolific author of a series of works that described, elaborated and refined the ideas of Hippocrates and other Greek physicians. Nonetheless, a clear definition of cancer eluded him, and he confused the characteristics of tumours with those of all kinds of other inflammations, including piles, abdominal swellings and fluid-filled cysts. When he did formulate a description – 'swellings which are contrary to nature and affect the whole body or any part of it' – it was so general that it was meaningless.

Galen's view of the mechanism of the disease was equally confused, as he believed that all health and illness was caused by the interaction of the four bodily humours, blood, phlegm, and yellow and black bile, the prevailing theory of the time. Tumours would grow, he argued, when the black bile responsible for the melancholic temperament became corrupted and stagnant. He suggested that this might happen when the spleen – the organ to the left side of the stomach beneath the diaphragm – failed to purify food toxins from the blood; Egyptians were supposedly at particular risk because they lived on ass's meat. Galen also suggested that old age was a factor: when the lively blood of youth became sluggish and stale, the black bile of older women resisted natural expulsion and collected in the breasts. Recommending a change in diet in favour of bloodless white meat, he also favoured bloodletting with leeches, and treated superficial cancers with the application of coal tar and caustic creams. Tumours that sat deep within the body were mostly not detected, and those that were in the cervix for instance were generally left untreated for fear of harming the patient.

'I have done as much for medicine as the Emperor Trajan did for the Roman Empire when he built bridges and roads through Italy,' Galen once boasted, and for a millennium his ideas dominated the Byzantine world under Islam and the great medical schools of Northern Italy; during the Renaissance his works were republished in more than 500 editions. Of course, many of Galen's theories were wrong, as he had been limited by the Roman belief that the human body was sacrosanct and could not be disturbed after death, and so he had little first-hand knowledge of the simplest human biological mechanisms. The only windows into human anatomy were through gladiators' wounds, while they were still alive.

Despite these limitations, the threads of Galen's influence reach towards us: the false but surprisingly pervasive notion, for instance, that cancer is caused by sadness has its roots in the idea that the melancholic humour was a determining factor. Similarly, he recommended that doctors adopt a formal and authoritative bedside manner in order that they could better win the trust of patients, a mode of behaviour which continues to be enacted in many consulting rooms.

However, medicine required the free-thinking men of

the Scientific Revolution to overturn the false ideas of the ancients.

§

My lifelong fear for Dad's health sprang, in part, from his inability to see his body as anything other than a rather pointless and badly engineered vessel to transport his brain. Blind to his own physicality, he hardly ate for reasons other than taste, nor did he exercise, and he smoked the odd cigar in the face of my mother's protests and drank copious amounts of red wine. His own mechanics continued to function regardless, apart from one occasion when I was about eight and I watched from an upstairs window as paramedics carried him, crying with back pain, into the ambulance. He soon healed.

Freed from the burden of having to think about his body, Dad could concentrate on developing his mind. Though his job had been to teach statistics at the University of Birmingham, he preferred to invigorate the imagination of his students by talking about the Romantic poets, Greek philosophers and eighteenth-century thinkers. Dad thought that those who simply wanted to learn the curriculum, would be better off reading the textbooks. Since retiring from teaching, his study of statistics had been demoted in favour of a broad range of other subjects – opera, history and Egyptian hieroglyphics among them.

His dominant passion was printing beautiful pamphlets and ephemera. For years, the garage of the family home had been filled with enormous cast-iron printing machines, the loft above it packed with hundreds of cases containing tiny lead letters and enormous wooden poster-type a foot high. As a child I often sat on the workbench watching him set the type by hand, roll the ink across the press and then feed in the paper, while the cast-iron press clattered like an old train. He was particularly proud of *Diseases of Printers*, a sixteen-page pamphlet in which he had reprinted a portion of a book first published in 1700 by Bernardino Ramazzini, the father of occupational health. This particular extract enumerated the various ailments that afflict 'servants to the republic of letters'. On its last page, Ramazzini advises that printers who are 'attacked by acute diseases must be treated with remedies that suit their particular case'.

&.

The first roots of this scientific medicine, which would eventually form the foundation of all cancer treatments, were planted in the second half of the sixteenth century, when anatomists began to dissect human bodies, and draw and describe the structure of each organ. Thus observation began to triumph over superstition. The first meaningful discovery of this scientific revolution was William Harvey's description, in 1628, of blood circulating around the body and travelling through both ventricles of the heart. Soon afterwards, other scientists began to understand the lymphatic system, a branching network of tubes that carries a colourless watery fluid called 'lymph' and a variety of glandular products. Discoveries about the digestion and the workings of the nerves quickly followed. The idea of the human body as an integrated engine was being slowly imprinted on to the minds of scientists.

The understanding of anatomy, however, had little immediate effect on the treatment of cancer; nor did the beautifully engraved pictures of the body's architecture give any real sense of how diseases could begin, develop and kill. In any case, cancer continued to kill comparatively tiny numbers. Some tumours were so out of the ordinary that in 1669 the family of a Dorset girl called Elizabeth Trevers – she of 'fair complexion, brown hair'd' – allowed thousands of strangers to inspect her enormously swollen breast, according to a report presented to the Royal Society in London. Similarly, Bernardino Ramazzini's exhaustive 600-page manual of occupational diseases, published in 1700, mentions cancer only once, stating that it affected the breasts of nuns: 'you can seldom find a convent that does not harbour this accursed pest, cancer, within its walls'.

During the seventeenth century, cancer remained a rare disease of older women, with little innovation in treatments. Instead, old methods were used: tumours were coated with poultices, plantain leaves, tobacco plants, arsenic pastes, the juices of the leaves of black nightshade, or lead and mercury tinctures; in the case of ulceration, rotten apples, frogspawn, fresh veal, or even pigeon, cut up when still alive, were applied. One popular treatment was to lay crawfish or crabs on the tumours, following the Doctrine of Signatures – the idea that nature itself would indicate the most appropriate treatment – which was a commonly held belief, and widely circulated in such books as Nicholas Culpeper's *The English Physician Enlarged* of 1653.

Surgery was rarely contemplated, as the incisions turned gangrenous and putrefied. When there was no other option, 'the surgeon should therefore be steadfast,' advised one teacher, 'and not allow himself to become disconcerted by the cries of the patient'. An ingenious Dutchman invented a device that looks to modern eyes like a giant cigar-cutter: two great semi-circular pincers made of good steel to hold the breast in place while a curved blade sliced it off in one movement, probably resulting in a very bloody wound that was likely to become gangrenous. Unsurprisingly, the device never became part of usual surgical practice.

❧

Dad had been suffering from a pain, which had developed from a dull throb to a jagged pierce, for three weeks when he first told me. His doctor had prescribed him a few pain-killers and had made an appointment for an X-ray. Active, and aged 72, he thought it so insignificant that he mentioned it only as an afterthought, in a telephone conversation.

A few weeks later, when I returned home for a Sunday lunch, Dad was cooking, chopping vegetables determinedly. It was the middle of April 2002. He was stooped, his shoulders were a little more rounded than usual, and his head had retreated into his shoulders. Instead of charging around the kitchen as was his way, he was sitting on a high stool. I asked how he was; he said he had a little back pain. I presumed that the cause was that he had been lifting the enormous cases of lead type for printing. But during lunch, when he could not move the casserole or plates, I realised the seriousness of his pain. He explained how during the previous few days he had been unable to sleep horizontally, and instead he had been fitfully sleeping in an armchair. Waiting on the result of the X-ray, he had been taking handfuls of painkillers. When his sister, Helen, heard about his self-medication she warned him as a doctor that he was close to overdosing.

⋅⋅⋅

Cancer began to become a little more visible in the middle of the eighteenth century. In about 1750, the first hospital dedicated solely to the disease opened in Rheims, in France, sponsored by the cathedral's cardinal – perhaps in order to care for his nuns. Yet medicine had little to offer cancer patients, despite leaps of insight being made in other areas of scientific endeavour, such as the description of the cosmos or the properties of gases. Fundamental questions remained unanswered: how was cancer to be distinguished from other swellings, such as those of leprosy? Was a tumour the symptom of the failure of the body as a whole, or just a specific organ? And, most important, what caused it? Filling the place of the facts was speculation. One theory, dating from the sixteenth century and widely believed throughout Europe, was that tumours were caused by 'acrimony', a process whereby chemicals apparently mixed in the blood. So convinced was one physician that he placed a sliver of excised breast tumour on his tongue in order to demonstrate that it was acidic. Others believed that tumours were the result of physical trauma, and one prudish physician suggested that the bawdy practice of touching women's breasts might lead to the disease. Some supposed that deep sorrow or shock was the cause.

Glimmers of enlightenment came with the publication, in 1761, of *De sedibus et causis morborum* (*On the Sites and Causes of Disease*), by Battista Morgagni, an 80-year-old professor of anatomy at the University of Padua. Drawing on the findings of more than 700 autopsies, he showed how the degeneration of certain organs was associated with certain diseases. He divided his book into four sections, covering diseases of the head, the chest, the abdomen, as well as surgical conditions. He described in detail the case history of each patient and the autopsy results, drawing links between these two sets of observations. He discovered that clots around the heart, for instance, had killed the patient with a heart attack; and he showed that a stroke had been caused by a change in the blood vessels in the head rather than to the flesh of the brain itself. Though he had little to say about cancer, Morgagni had created a new method, pathology, to understand how diseases progressed. Shifting medicine's focus away from symptoms and towards the deterioration of specific organs, he created a tool as profound as Galileo's telescope, which had opened up the heavens.

੪

The day after Dad cooked Sunday lunch, I sent him lists of chiropractors and osteopaths, convinced that a little manipulation would end the pain. When they demanded to see X-rays, he pursued his GP for the results. The following day, Dad was called to the surgery. The image was clear: one of his neck vertebrae had crumbled. A second seemed to be cracking.

The doctor had organised an emergency hospital admission, and Dad walked the mile to get there. His neck was so fragile that had he tripped then, he would have died. At the hospital he was placed on the bed of the magnetic resonance imaging scanner. Once in the humming sarcophagus of the machine, a pain of an intensity he had never experienced before seared through his neck. Later he realised that it was the second vertebrae collapsing.

For a man who had spent so much of his life defining himself through his intellect, there seemed to be something particularly malicious about the way that nature was now trying to disconnect his head from the rest of his body. It was as if, after years of being ignored, his physical self was now reasserting itself with a bold, new certainty.

ఄ

A century after Isaac Newton had transformed the physical sciences, cancer medicine was, at last, beginning to develop equally rapidly. In 1775, Sir Percival Pott of St Bartholomew's Hospital, in London, realised that chimney sweeps were often on his wards with scrotal cancer. As boys they had been 'thrust up narrow, sometimes hot, chimnies where they are burned and almost suffocated,' he wrote. 'When they get to puberty they become particularly liable to a most noisome, painful and fatal disease.' It was the first identification of an industrial cancer. And by blaming the soot, he was the first to propose that chemicals could cause the disease, albeit for a very specific and rare tumour. At the same time, cancer was becoming more visible, so much so that, in 1791, the brewer Samuel Whitbread endowed the first cancer ward in London, at the Middlesex Hospital.

Nonetheless, tuberculosis, and epidemics including dysentery, typhus and cholera, dominated the public's imagination at the beginning of the nineteenth century, because cancer was still quite rare. The first statistical analysis of deaths from cancer was carried out by Domenico Antonio Rigoni-Stern in Verona between 1760 and 1839. During that time, 994 women and only 142 men had died of the disease in that city. In total, less than one death per hundred was due to the disease. Today the equivalent figure is about 25 per cent – or one in four deaths – some of the increase owing to better diagnosis and our lengthening lifespans.

However, the disease was becoming so worrisome that, in 1802, a group of Scottish worthies thought it necessary to gather together with the 'intention being solely that of cooperating in the laudable endeavour to lessen the mals of human misery, by calling for the assistance of others by exerting themselves to obtain remedy for a most painful and dreadful disease, against which all medicine and methods of treatment hitherto proposed and tried have been unavailing'. Although they understood that this was a disease that predominantly affected old people, they had few other insights. So they published a brochure in order to inspire men of letters to address this difficult problem, asking a series of questions: Is cancer a primary disease? Is it hereditary? Is it contagious? Is there a temperament of the body more susceptible? Can it be cured naturally? And do 'brute creatures' also suffer? Four years later, there was little to report by way of answers.

One reason for the lack of progress was a shortage of bodies for dissection throughout Europe and America. Many families refused to have their loved ones' souls disturbed; others were afraid that scientists would turn cadavers into monsters – just as in Mary Shelley's best-selling *Frankenstein*, published in 1818. In desperation, anatomists retained the services of bodysnatchers to dig up graves and cart the rotting remains to medical schools. Most famously, William Burke and William Hare from Edinburgh murdered their victims before selling them. In 1827, this rising conflict between the public and the dissectors – who saw themselves as the heralds of a new age of science – spilled on to the streets. In Aberdeen, 20,000 people gathered outside the medical school; as their numbers swelled, the gates gave way and soon relatives of the deceased ran through the corridors, fighting with doctors and carrying off the bodies of their friends and relatives. There had already been a riot in New York, sparked when a medical student taunted a young boy, claiming that a dismembered arm belonged to his mother.

By 1832, British and North American legislatures were therefore forced to pass 'Anatomy Acts', which regulated dissection, while insisting that workhouses release the bodies of the destitute to medical research. Scientists were, for the first time, able to dissect thousands of cadavers to investigate the natural history of diseases. Cancer had a unique position in these researchers' plans, because doctors rightly assumed that studying the unregulated growth of tumours might give them insights into how normal flesh developed. So, as the new age of cancer science began, doctors set out to understand not only one of humanity's most pernicious threats but also the secrets of human life itself.

Surgery:
the bloody butchery

O N SATURDAY 9 APRIL 1831, a year before the passage of the Anatomy Act, but a few months after the opening of the world's first purpose-built passenger railway, a crowd of men in top hats and coat-tails showed their 'hospital tickets' and entered the operating theatre of Guy's Hospital in London. Hundreds of others jostled on the street outside. An attempt had already been made by the hospital authorities to prevent a scrum by moving the date forward by three days, but the tight, gossiping community of London's doctors had defeated the ruse.

The patient in question was a 32-year-old Chinese labourer called Hoo Loo, who had disembarked at the Royal Docks from a sailing ship, a so-called East Indiaman, with some difficulty three weeks previously. He was carrying an enormous tumour four feet in circumference, which hung from his lower abdomen, enveloping his penis, to below his knees. It was 'of a nature and extent hitherto unseen in this country'. Although the size of Hoo Loo's growth made it exceptional, lumps, boils and malignancies were often seen to disfigure the human form in the age before routine surgery. Hoo Loo's had been growing for ten years, but his doctors in Canton had refused him treatment. Because it had continued to grow, he had travelled for six months to London in the belief that there the art of surgery was somewhat more advanced and that the profession would have no such qualms in operating on him. On arriving at Guy's Hospital he must have been aware of the excitement, for as he lay waiting for the operation his days were interrupted by 'a great number of persons of all ranks' keen to examine this oriental curiosity.

Because of the swelling crowds, it was announced that the operation was to be held in the 'Great Anatomical Theatre'. A 'tremendous rush' ensued as 680 gentlemen pushed their way into the auditorium. Fifteen minutes later, Hoo Loo was carried in and laid on the dissecting table, which was still stained black with blood from previous guests. Two nurses tied his limbs to the table so that he would not be able to flinch from pain – there being no such thing as anaesthesia then – and Hoo Loo looked on, seeming to contemplate the operation with a fortitude 'never exceeded in the annals of surgery'. The nurses then covered his face so that he might not see the imminent procedure.

Then entered Sir Astley Cooper, the greatest physician of his day, renowned for helping to embalm the body of King George IV, for stealing a dog for the purpose of vivisection and for having boasted to a parliamentary committee of his close relationship with bodysnatchers. Having been reprimanded once for arriving at the royal chamber wearing a morning coat still covered in someone else's viscera, he was probably similarly attired on the day of Hoo Loo's operation. Together with the surgeon, Charles Key, he decided that the operation should attempt to preserve the genital organs.

Mr Key stationed himself in front of the tumour and made the first incision just below the right side of Hoo Loo's abdomen. With barely a groan or a gasp from the patient, Key continued for six inches down the right-hand side of the penis and around the tumour. 'The quality which is considered of the highest order in surgical operations, is self possession,' Sir Cooper had once lectured. 'The head must always direct the hand.' Key repeated the manoeuvre on the patient's left side, connecting the two cuts below the base of the penis. Then Key lifted the tumour up, and cut around the urethra. The audience was silent, craning to see and hear Hoo Loo. Cutting veins, Key reached for silk threads to tie them, possibly holding the bloodied scalpel in his teeth, as was the practice. The patient 'firmly set his teeth and resignedly strung every nerve in obedience to the determination with which he had first submitted to the knife'. After each incision, Hoo Loo was given some time to recover from the 'fits of exhaustion', as without anaesthetic the trauma of the knife was often almost as dangerous as the cuts themselves. Then, with 'great neatness', Key attempted to cut around the penis in order to separate the tumour. As more than a hour had passed since the first incision, Cooper began to worry that its protraction was detrimental to the patient, most other operations being over in a few minutes. So he insisted that the operation be completed as quickly as possible by sacrificing the genitals.

Hoo Loo was drifting in and out of consciousness. The nurses rubbed his toes and injected brandy into his stomach in a bid to keep him awake. But already a pint of Hoo Loo's blood had been lost, some of it congealing around the operating table. Students in the audience offered to give their own blood for Hoo Loo's life, and a transfusion of a quarter of a pint had been attempted. Key continued to cut and, one hour and forty minutes after beginning, he freed the tumour from the body. It weighed fifty-eight pounds. With a final gasp, Hoo Loo collapsed into unconsciousness. The doctors sensed his heart 'gradually and perceptibly' sinking. Then he died.

The following week, the medical journal *The Lancet* criticised the surgeons for killing Hoo Loo, reasoning that his operation had taken place too early – before he had the opportunity to acclimatise to the British weather – and because his vital force had been constricted by the lack of air in the room. In the following weeks, its correspondence columns also criticised Sir Astley Cooper's recklessness. 'I think that this operation could neither advance science of surgery,' wrote W. Simpson of Hammersmith, 'nor be otherwise beneficial to the human race; that it was neither sanctioned by reason, nor warranted by experience.'

Hoo Loo was an extreme example of the brutality, and often futility, of surgery in the early nineteenth century. Even the relatively simple excision of a breast tumour created a 'terror that surpasses all description & the most torturing pain,' wrote the novelist Fanny Burney. 'When the dreadful steel was plunged into my breast – cutting through the veins, arteries, flesh, nerves – I needed no injunctions not to restrain my cries. I began a scream that lasted un-intermittingly during the whole time of the incision – & I marvel that it rings not in my ears still!' In general, operations were to be avoided, and were only carried out when a tumour had become so enlarged or was bleeding so profusely that it was imminently threatening life. And of course, without any techniques to see inside the body, surgeons contemplated only tumours on the surface of the skin, or at the very most in the cervix.

As well as the pain, the other reason for the reluctance to operate on tumours was that those patients who did not die on the table often succumbed shortly afterwards to a range of 'hospital diseases', the symptoms of which were rotting surgical wounds and rising bodily temperatures. Following the illness of a single patient, the hospital air would turn foul until patients in the neighbouring beds, and then in other wards, would all fall ill. Some scientists speculated that the cause of this terror was 'spontaneous generation', in which the mixing fluids of the body were causing self-destruction. To guard against this eventuality, leeches were applied to the healing wounds. But nothing seemed to reduce the numbers of fatalities. The trouble was, of course, that nobody really understood how hospital diseases developed and spread, and therefore no one knew the precautions to take against them.

❧

At 8.30, the morning after his admission, Dad was pushed on a trolley through the corridors of the Queen Elizabeth Hospital in Birmingham – not far from the rooms where my sister and I were born. I was in London, because although Mum had left a message to say that Dad was in hospital, I had no inkling that he was about to undergo emergency surgery. On entering through the double doors of the grey utilitarian theatre, Dad saw his surgeon, Mr Graham Flint. Dad had long derided the affectation of English surgeons calling themselves Mister, or Miss, rather than Doctor as is the case in America. The distinction had been created in the seventeenth century, he argued, when surgeons had been skilled craftsmen as opposed to university-trained doctors, but he thought there was no need for its continuance. But he was in no position to remonstrate. Also in the theatre were a nurse, a runner and an anaesthetist. Dad had been told that the surgery would stabilise his neck. Without it he would become paralysed and incontinent and remain in great pain. As all the forces of life – blood, air and nerves – travel through the neck, he also knew there was a risk that the surgery might initiate what it was intended to forestall.

❧

In 1846, fifteen years after the Hoo Loo debacle, steamships were breaking the ocean waves, railways were snaking across England, and the newly coined word 'scientist' was in much use among London's recently formed learned societies.

The callow 27-year-old William Thomas Green Morton was putting his finishing touches to his inhaler for ether, in

Boston, Massachusetts. The chemical had been discovered centuries earlier, but had thus far been used only for entertainment – for ether-frolics, evenings of enjoyable intoxication. A dentist, entrepreneur and inventor, Morton had dreamt up the idea of the ether inhaler in order to save his patients from pain – and in the febrile hope that he would make his fortune. As ether was widely available and someone else had noticed its analgesic qualities, Morton was fearful that others would steal his idea, so he called the magic compound 'Letheon' to disguise its rather simple origin. He had tested it on a spaniel and on one of his assistants. For wider recognition, he had persuaded the eminent surgeon John Collins Warren of the Massachusetts General Hospital to allow a demonstration of the device on a real patient. However, Morton's wife, Elizabeth, had little enthusiasm for the event, 'for the strongest influences had been brought to bear upon me to dissuade him from making the attempt,' she said. 'It did not seem possible that so young a man … could be wiser than the learned and scientific men before whom he proposed to make the demonstration.' She was worried that he would be ridiculed, or that he would kill the patient and be tried for manslaughter.

At the appointed time, on 16 October 1846, a 20-year-old painter from Boston called Gilbert Abbott settled into a chair in the operating theatre, a vascular tumour protruding from his neck. A crowd of doctors had gathered for the demonstration. But after fifteen minutes of waiting for Morton, Dr Warren said derisively, 'I presume he is otherwise engaged', and laughed. Perhaps it was the argument with his wife that had delayed Morton. But just as the surgeon was picking up his scalpel, Morton arrived. 'Your patient is ready,' said Dr Warren. Morton pulled out a glass flask containing sponges soaked in 'Letheon'. Abbott fastened his lips to the mouthpiece and sucked the ether-saturated air into his lungs. Within a few minutes, the patient was asleep. '*Your* patient is ready,' Morton said to the surgeon. One of the onlookers, a doctor called Washington Ayer, described that moment as 'the most sublime scene ever witnessed in an operating theatre'.

The first cut was two or three inches long, 'to my great surprise without any starting, crying or other indication of pain,' said Warren. Separating the veins that passed through the tumour, he tied them with silk thread. As the wound was being sewn up, Abbott flailed his limbs and uttered 'extraordinary expressions'. On completing the operation, Warren turned to the onlookers and said, 'Gentlemen, this is no humbug.' It was the first public demonstration of anaesthesia. When Abbott awoke, he explained that though he had felt no pain, he had felt the draw of the blade as if it were a blunt instrument across his neck.

Within days, newspapers were reporting the success. The *People's Journal* in London crowed, 'WE HAVE CONQUERED PAIN. This is indeed a glorious victory to announce. A victory of pure intellect ... It is a victory not for today, not for our own time, but for another age, and all time – not for one nation, but for all nations, from generation to generation, as long as the world shall last.'

The success of Gilbert Abbott's surgery spread anaesthesia around the world. Malignant lumps and tumours could now be excised without terrorising the patient; however, most patients remained reluctant to go under the knife because of the fear and danger of hospital diseases, and the putrefaction of their wounds.

❧

Before the surgery began, Dad stared up at the ceiling of the operating theatre wondering if he would ever see the light again; whether he would be able to see his beloved grandchildren or touch his printing machines once more. Pads were applied to his chest to measure his heart beat; a device was placed on his finger to test for the amount of oxygen in his blood; and a cuff was placed around his arm to monitor his blood pressure. A tube was inserted into his mouth to keep his airways free. A mask was placed over his mouth. A needled end of a tube was pushed into a vein in the back of his hand. The anaesthetist asked Dad if he was ready, and injected a drug into his hand. Later, Dad told me he had momentarily hallucinated, seeing spiders crawling across the ceiling. He remembered nothing more.

❧

In 1867, twenty years after the birth of anaesthesia, telegraph machines chattered in every post office; steam drove printing machines and ironworks; and a debate raged about Charles Darwin's idea that man was created by nature, not God.

A 44-year-old Londoner called Isabella Pim discovered a large lump growing in her breast that June. As the daughter of the scientist Joseph Jackson Lister, who had radically improved the compound microscope in 1830, she went to see one of the city's most renowned doctors, James Paget of Wimpole Street. But he explained that the dangers of surgery were too great, because the cancer had progressed so far. Unwilling to accept such a bleak prognosis, she travelled to Edinburgh to see James Syme, her brother's father-in-law and a well-known physician, for a second opinion; he also recommended inaction. Both were concerned about the problem of hospital diseases, which killed so many patients.

Before seeking the advice of a quack, she went to her brother, Joseph Lister, the professor of surgery at the Glasgow Royal Infirmary. Just three months earlier he had published a series of articles in *The Lancet* that contained some of the most significant research of the age. In them he had described how he had improved the chances of survival for patients who had suffered fractures of the bone that had punctured the skin. While previously about half of such patients would die of hospital diseases, ten out of eleven of Lister's survived, the other dying of haemorrhage rather than infection.

Lister's breakthrough was founded on a new under-standing of the mechanism of disease. Two years previously, he had read a scientific paper by the then unknown Louis Pasteur, who had shown that minute, seemingly inanimate particles that were suspended in the air were, in fact, the germs of various low forms of life. Lister applied this abstract scientific insight to hospital diseases, surmising that they too were caused by 'germs'. Preventing these from entering the wound or collecting nearby, therefore, became the central tenet of what was soon known as the Listerian method. A dilute solution of carbolic acid was to be sprayed in the air of the operating theatre, soaked into the lint of dressings and used to clean the scalpel and forceps. When his sister sought his advice, the method had thus far been used only to treat abscesses and complex fractures.

The lump in his sister's breast threw Lister into a dilemma. Although he was convinced of his own method, other doctors had doubted it. Were his critics correct, an operation on his sister might curtail rather than extend her life. So he too travelled to Edinburgh to consult his father-in-law, James Syme. 'No one can say that the operation does not afford a chance,' offered Syme. Perhaps his change of heart was the result of his own recent experiments with the Listerian method. 'I felt his true kindness and *manifest*, though little expressed, sympathy, very much and left Edinburgh very much relieved,' wrote Lister.

Although Lister had done a number of tumour excisions, he took the precaution of practising the operation on a corpse. 'I suppose before this reaches thee the operation of darling B[ella] will be over,' wrote Lister on 16 June to his father. Apprehensive of operating on his own family, he continued, 'It is very satisfactory to me that B seems to have thorough confidence in me. She distinctly says she would much rather have me to perform the operation than anyone else. And considering *what* the operation is to be I would rather not let anyone else do it.'

The following day, his sister lay on the table in Lister's house in Woodside Place in Glasgow. We 'saw how much it cost him to undertake so bold a procedure for the first time on one so dear to him,' said Hector Cameron, who was assisting. Two nurses were also present. Bella's breast was wiped down with carbolic acid, a lint soaked in it was placed over the area of the operation, and Lister also dipped his scalpel in the acid. She breathed in chloroform, considered to be an advancement on ether, and was soon asleep. Lister gingerly lifted the lint and cut a large incision in her breast. Breast incisions are usually bloody, and he staunched the flow by burning the flesh, closing the smaller blood vessels in the process. He cut around the larger blood vessels that connected the tumour to the body, tied them with silk thread, then severed them. The whole procedure was undertaken as if by a seamstress unpicking a garment of enormous complexity. The threads that bound the tumour to the body, each blood vessel and lymph duct, were sealed and then cut in this way. Eventually the lump was freed from the body. Those blood vessels that had been close to the tumour, but remained with the body, he stripped clean of flesh for fear of leaving malignant remnants. Afterwards, when the wound had been sewn up, the lint was replaced. The following day, Lister wrote to his father, 'I may say that the operation was at least as well as if she had not been my sister. But I do not wish to do such a thing again.' In the days that followed, the wound did not turn septic.

Seven weeks after the operation, Lister went to Dublin to present a paper at a British Medical Association meeting. Whereas previously he had advocated his technique for fractures and abscesses, now he presented it as a general method, 'On the Antiseptic Principle in the Practice of Surgery'. Since he had started using it himself, he declared, not a single case of hospital gangrene had appeared on his wards. 'As there appears to be no doubt regarding the cause of this change, the important fact can hardly be exaggerated.'

Lister's detractors filled the columns of the medical press in the following weeks. 'Where are these little beasts? Show them us, and we shall believe in them. Has anyone seen them yet?' asked one. But Lister was a formidable opponent, touring Europe and America and telling anyone who would listen about his method that stopped patients from dying. His own sister did not die from the operation, and lived for three more years before she succumbed to a secondary cancer of the liver.

During the following two decades, versions of the Listerian method were adopted by most doctors. Operating gowns, rubber gloves, sparkling cleanliness and the demise of the surgeon's audience all added to safety. Gambling with the surgeon's knife was becoming progressively less risky.

§.

Dad's surgeon, Graham Flint, and the other staff were gowned and gloved; their scalpels were sterile, the needles were new. Dad lay on his back. Flint positioned my father's head on a pillow. Years of experience had taught him not to push the head too far back because although this revealed the neck, it also tightened the throat, making it more difficult to manipulate during the operation. A nurse disinfected Dad's skin. Flint took a scalpel and cut for six or seven centimetres, in a line that ran from Dad's right collarbone towards his ear. With some force, Flint pushed Dad's voice box to one side and the carotid artery in the other direction. Through the cavity, he could now see the shape of Dad's spine, surrounded by fine muscles.

§.

In 1881, fifty years after Hoo Loo's operation, a 43-year-old woman called Therese Heller was admitted to the clinic of the great surgeon Theodor Billroth, in Vienna. Suffering from indigestion, she found eating food painful, and vomited regularly. She was pale, her pulse was weak and, for six weeks, she had been losing weight as her only nourishment was buttermilk. Now she had retired to bed, where her eight children were forced to look after her. When Billroth pressed her stomach he felt a fist-size tumour resting just beneath the skin.

Fat and fifty years old, Billroth was greatly concerned with how history would judge him. This anxiety made him self-destructively depressed, especially when he compared himself to his good friend Johannes Brahms, who he thought had the power to compose sublime, everlasting music. For 'some small compensation for my vexation', Billroth decided that Therese Heller would be the experimental subject of an ambitious operation that would excise a small section of her stomach and then rejoin the healthy parts of the digestive tract, much as one would cut out a small part of a pipe and then rejoin the ends. For the previous four years Billroth had been preparing for this moment by experimenting on dogs' stomachs to see how surgical wounds heal even in the presence of gastric juices. Though others had attempted this operation, their patients had all quickly died.

Four days after her first consultation, Therese Heller was wheeled into the operating theatre. Billroth's team had been trained to work like an engine; they kept the room at a constant 24° C, administered a mixture of ether, alcohol and chloroform and swabbed her belly with carbolic acid. 'There was not the slightest confusion,' said Billroth, 'not a minute of unnecessary delay.' Billroth's first incision was a deft three-inch cut above her navel. The tumour was revealed, above and slightly to the right of the umbilicus, the size of a 'medium sized apple'. Having separated the tumour from the nerves and blood vessels, he lifted the tumour and stomach through the abdominal wound, a nurse placing a large sponge beneath it for support. The tumour encircled the fleshy tubing of the gut. Next Billroth made an incision above the tumour, across the lower half of the stomach, and an incision below it, through the upper end of the duodenum. The tumour was then removed, together with the lower half of the stomach to which it was attached. Finally he sewed the clean end of the stomach to the top of the intestine, as if he were attaching two ends of pipe together, and stitched up her abdomen. An hour and a half after he had begun, her wound was wiped with carbolic acid and dressed.

After the operation, Heller suffered no weakness or pain. 'I was happily surprised,' wrote Billroth after six days, 'by her entirely smooth course.' Nursed back to strength on hourly buttermilk, within a few days she demanded to be moved to a larger ward because she was bored. Fourteen days later, Billroth wrote excitedly to a friend that she remained in good spirits: 'I hardly wish to hazard a belief that everything will continue so smoothly.'

Unfortunately, the tumour recurred and, after eighty-four days, Therese Heller died. Though disappointed, Billroth did not see this as a sign of failure but repeated the operation and reported the results excitedly.

The technical prowess of the Victorian age had at last reached the operating theatre. The human body, it seemed, was a machine every bit as susceptible to repair as the steam engine or the typewriter. And Billroth's operation had demonstrated that even cancers hidden deep within the body could be susceptible to surgery. In the coming years, it became possible to excise tumours from such places as the oesophagus, the bowels and the bladder.

❧

Looking through Dad's neck wound, Flint saw there was some inflammation around the spinal cord. Working with an X-ray image that showed the exact position of the spinal collapse, Flint cut away the fine spinal muscles to reveal the disease. The bone was not solid but flecked through with particles of fleshy redness. Surrounding the tumour was a network of specially built blood vessels. Dad was losing blood, but Flint sucked it away with a straw-like device – by the end of the operation he had lost about 700 ml, roughly the same amount as Hoo Loo. Now Flint chipped away at the two diseased vertebrae, excising the two links from the chain of bones that had made Dad's spine.

The focus of the operation moved to Dad's hip. Flint cut it open and hammered out a fragment of bone a few centimetres in length. He placed this fragment in Dad's neck between the two healthy vertebrae. Over it, he placed a titanium pillar. At both ends, Flint twisted two inch-long screws to anchor it to the bones. The idea was that in time the bone would grow back, but that until then the scaffolding would support Dad's head. Two and a half hours later, Dad was wheeled back on to the ward.

Two days after surgery, Dad lay on his back in a hospital bed. The ward was noisy, and the agony of other patients seemed to echo through the corridors. His pillow was smeared with blood. The back of his head was a mass of matted hair. 'My head is bloody but unbowed,' he said, quoting the Victorian poet W. E. Henley. Fearful that he might be close to death, I had written a letter saying I loved him – something I had never told him before – which I handed to him. Dad was already asking me questions about the history of medicine, about how Victorian surgery had developed. He told me what he knew about the history of cancer, talking until he was parched and red in the face, as if the ability to impart knowledge was his affirmation that he was alive.

The next day, I wandered along the hospital corridor. My first sight was of his empty bed. I thought he had died in the night. But as I turned the corner, I saw him sitting up in a chair, and in good spirits. Alive, he knew he was lucky.

Even though he was recovering, we had not been told what had caused the collapse in the first place.

Cells:

a scientific revolution

IN MARCH 1845, a 50-year-old cook called Marie Straide was admitted to the Charité Hospital in Berlin with swollen legs, a painful stomach and bleeding diarrhoea. Doctors prodded her aching abdomen, but they had no idea what she was suffering from nor how to treat it. By May, an acute pain had emerged in her spleen. In June, her nose bled severely and repeatedly. The doctors injected her with a salt of potassium and aluminium called 'alum' and made her drink a special preparation of sulphur because they believed it would strengthen her blood. But her decline continued.

To understand her disease, the doctors studied Karl Rokitansky's *Handbuch der Pathologischen Anatomie* (*A Manual of Pathological Anatomy*), which had been published in two volumes during the previous three years and was the most comprehensive taxonomy to date. Rokitansky had classified many diseases, from tumours and tuberculosis to smallpox and cirrhosis, matching their symptoms to the discoloration, inflammation and decay of various organs. Each dysfunction of the body was lovingly described in picturesque language – degenerated viscera, for example, was likened to 'raspberry jelly', 'a purée of peas' or 'coffee grounds'.

Although encyclopaedic, the *Manual* was not in any sense an innovation as the ideas underpinning pathology had been created more than fifty years previously. Rokitansky had simply added detail to an existing body of knowledge by collating the results of more than ten thousand autopsies that he had carried out during the previous fifteen years as the professor of pathology in Vienna. Equally, the *Manual* did not reflect the current state of science. In some sections, Rokitansky described mysterious blood-borne substances that caused disease, as if he still held Galenic ideas. At the same time, he had never used a microscope, a technology that had been significantly improved since he had begun work, when their crude lenses had produced distorted images which were fringed in refracted rainbows. By the time Marie Straide arrived at the Charité Hospital, it had become possible, however, to grind two lenses so that they magnified clearly by more than a hundred times. These optical discoveries had been made in 1830, by Joseph Jackson Lister – a London scientist and the father of Joseph Lister and Isabella Pim. Nonetheless, Rokitansky had preferred to use his naked eyes. The resulting *Manual* was therefore not only a partial description of the workings of the diseased body, but also somewhat archaic.

So although Marie Straide's doctors searched, they found no series of cases which exactly paralleled her symptoms. With little idea of what was going on beneath her skin, it was as if they saw the hands moving past the hours on a timepiece but had no inklings of the internal mechanism causing the movement.

On 21 July, four and half months after she had arrived at the hospital, Marie Straide's doctors feared her imminent death, and made deep cuts in Straide's hands in an attempt to drain away the vast amounts of pus that had collected. In any case, Marie Straide declined rapidly, like 'a small boat sinking in the waves', and ten days later she died. Twenty-eight hours after her death, she was laid out naked on the slab of Charité's 'death house'. A young trainee doctor called Rudolf Virchow stood beside her.

Rudolf Virchow was the son of the treasurer of a small town called Schivelbein, in the state of Pomerania, and had arrived in Berlin at the age of 18 to study medicine, driven by a ferocious ambition. Within a year of his graduation, some months previously, he had pushed aside the ageing director of the morgue, and now, at the age of 24, was responsible for the examination of all cadavers from the 1,500-bed hospital. Callow and arrogant, he believed that he was on the vanguard of a revolution that was destroying myth and superstition. 'Those were the days of great degeneration in medicine,' he later wrote. 'The method of orderly investigation had been completely lost … People found themselves in the hopeless ruins as the old systems collapsed; filled with exaggerated expectations, they seized on any fragment which a bold spectator might choose to cast out.'

The smell of the morgue was intensified by the summer's heat. Virchow began by sawing open the skull and examining the brain; it looked normal. He then moved to the right side of Marie Straide, his left hand nearest her head. Though other pathologists held scalpels like pencils, Virchow grasped his in the palm of his hand, rather like a butcher might hold a knife, so that he could make confident strokes. He cut down the length of her torso, from under her chin to her pubis.

Cutting through the sternum, he revealed her heart which contained 'greenish-yellow white clots'. Then he investigated her abdomen, discovering her spleen to be 'almost a foot long', four or five times the size of a healthy organ, and 'very dark brown-red and of timber-like consistency'.

Systematically opening up each organ and limb, he dictated to his assistants his findings. Finally he moved to the intestines. 'It is a disagreeable matter,' he later told his students. 'Even with the greatest care, one can scarcely avoid soiling oneself, the instruments and receptacles, the subject and the table on which it lies.' Virchow found nothing abnormal in Marie Straide's guts.

Each autopsy was executed in exactly the same way so that results could be compared. Every tiny observation, no matter how seemingly insignificant, was noted; case reports often ran to ten or more pages; examinations usually took almost three hours. As he carried out three or four a day, this meant he worked from eight in the morning to beyond midnight with only a short break for dinner. He complained that he was being paid less for a month's work than a young man on a railroad might earn in a day, but, he proudly wrote to his father, 'it is a truly Danaidean task, this medicine; nothing has been systematically studied. One must work through everything for oneself from the beginning, and this is so difficult that one at times loses heart.'

Where Virchow differed from pathologists of the previous generation, such as Rokitansky, was that at every stage of the autopsy, he placed slivers of flesh and smears of blood underneath a microscope. With the new greater resolution he could see that a mass of flesh that looked undifferentiated to the eye was, in fact, comprised of millions of tiny cells, each about one-hundredth of a millimetre in diameter. Each cell had a dark central spot, called the nucleus, which was surrounded by some kind of fluid, all of which was enclosed by a wall. Virchow was obsessed with this microscopic world, and an enthusiastic advocate of the so-called 'cell theory', which had been coined by others just six years before. In Virchow's formulation, this meant that 'Life is, in essence, cell activity.'

With each specimen from Marie Straide's body, Virchow adjusted the mirror beneath the microscope to catch the sun or the candlelight. He already knew that healthy blood looked mostly like a sea of small corpuscles, the so-called red blood cells, although their colour was diminished during magnification. He also knew that in healthy blood there were occasionally much larger and less regularly shaped corpuscles, the white blood cells. He found that Marie Straide's blood was full of these larger irregular white blood cells, some horseshoe in shape, some with clover-leaf nuclei. In each blood sample – from the heart, the hands and the spleen – the anomalous pattern repeated itself with the smaller red cells appearing only infrequently. In his report on the case, published three months after the autopsy, Virchow outlined what he later considered to be his first contribution to science: the classification of a hitherto unidentified disease resulting from a proliferation of white blood cells. Within a year, Virchow had written two more articles about 'white blood' and coined the term 'leukaemia' (*leukos* being the Greek word for 'white') to describe it. Today, it is understood to be a cancer of the blood.

❦

After Dad's operation, a lump a few centimetres across containing the collapsed vertebrae was placed in a small plastic tub and taken from the operating theatre to the histology laboratory, where acrid-smelling formalin was added. It seeped into the flesh, preventing putrefaction and the collapse of the cells' structures – 'fixing it', in the language of pathologists. Stacked up on the workbenches were other plastic pots, some almost as large as buckets, containing stomachs, breasts, lungs and various other human parts; all were being bathed for the requisite twenty-four hours.

The following day, when Dad was still groggy from the anaesthetic, a pathologist began what is called the 'cut-up'. Dad's tumour was placed on the draining surface. Thin slivers of flesh, the area of a stamp, the thickness of a pencil, were carefully cut away. Each was placed in a tiny plastic box, the perforated steel lids of which clicked shut. A basket of these numbered boxes was placed inside a so-called tissue processing machine, which rumbled and whirred overnight, bathing each sample in a variety of chemicals in order to remove their remaining moisture.

While Dad was recovering from his operation, his doctors told us that the lump in his neck was probably some kind of cancer. But there was no consensus on its origin. The tumour might have developed originally in his neck; or cells might have broken off from a primary tumour sited elsewhere in his body, and floated around the bloodstream until they reached the neck. With this uncertainty, the doctors advised patience. We all waited for a full report, hoping for some piece of information that would allow us to envisage a cure.

꘡

The day after Marie Straide's autopsy, Virchow made a speech in front of privy councillors, military doctors and the directors of the hospital, arguing for empirical observations, the microscope and systematic scientific practice. Writing to his father, he said that some criticised him for being 'new fangled', as many in the profession continued to believe in the old laws of apothecary, or in medical treatment based on medieval ideas about the body. Despite his harsh reception, Virchow remained confident and declared that his audience was even 'duller than I had previously supposed'.

During the following year, Virchow continued to classify diseases ranging from cysts on a finger's tendons to blockages of the pulmonary artery, and added his microscopic insights to the corpus of knowledge created by Rokitansky and others. But his real desire was to formulate, as Newton had in physics, the laws of human biology. 'It is the privilege of great men to find simple laws,' wrote Virchow. But he understood the problems of discovering such a universal rule: 'Only the simple is difficult to distinguish; the manifold, forming itself differently on all sides, is seen by ordinary eyes.' Nonetheless, Virchow searched for the underlying mechanism to explain how organs degraded, tumours grew and blood filled with white cells.

Karl Rokitansky addressed exactly these questions in a

third volume of his *Manual of Pathological Anatomy*, published some months after Marie Straide's death. Although the previous two volumes had concentrated on the classification of disease, now he boldly expounded a new theory: that all new growths were caused by the mixing of various components of a mysterious bodily fluid which he called the *blastema*. He explained that tumours miraculously appeared in the body just as crystals might spring from clear, colourless liquids. In each section of this volume of the *Manual*, he refined these ideas: brain tumours, for instance, were the 'silt' in the body's pipe work. The notion chimed with a theory that many doctors already held to be self-evident, that life emerged through 'spontaneous generation', as if by alchemy from its surrounding environment: thus mould developed from fruits, maggots from flesh and, why not, tumours from blood.

When Virchow – seventeen years Rokitansky's junior – read the latest volume he was overcome with sadness, remarking that he had rarely seen a work 'more dangerous to medicine'. Rokitansky's book 'blends its hypotheses so intimately with genuine observations of fact that a line of division can no longer be found,' claimed Virchow in a review published in the *Preussische Medizinal-Zeitung* in December 1846, echoing John Stuart Mill's warning to scientists, in his recently published *System of Logic*, about the dangers of formulating inaccurate theories grounded on limited data. Rokitansky had turned 'natural science into a system of articles of faith,' wrote Virchow, enumerating the errors, gaps and contradictions that had been created by an overactive mind. The idea of a *blastema* was particularly flawed, and Virchow had seen no traces of it when he had looked down microscopes; rather it seemed to be inspired by the notion that Galenic humours caused disease. Virchow declared the *blastema* to be a 'monstrous anachronism'.

Virchow was risking his career as a junior doctor by attacking the greatest work of pathology yet published. 'Now a great uproar has broken out,' he wrote soon afterwards. 'The young colleagues in Vienna are outraged.' Yet, the leading figures of the Berlin medical community immediately wrote articles of support, and Rokitansky soon realised his errors, erasing every mention of the *blastema* from the next edition of the *Manual*. At the end of his career, Virchow would proudly recall this moment as the last time that Galenic humours appeared in the 'scientific marketplace'.

꙳

A few days after Dad's operation, the samples of his flesh had been cut, fixed and dehydrated. The slivers of flesh were now sitting in the pathology laboratory each in a plastic case the size of a matchbox. They were next to a machine that kept paraffin wax molten. A technician opened the lid of one of the cases, checked that the fragile sliver of flesh was at its centre, and then placed it under the machine's nozzle so that wax could be poured into the case. In this way, each piece of flesh was embedded, like a fly in amber.

In another room, a technician placed one of these wax blocks on to a microtome, a slicing machine that looked like a smaller version of the ones used for ham in delicatessens. As the handle was turned, slivers of waxy flesh a few thousandths of a millimetre thick were cut off, the force of the steel wrinkling the soft wax of the samples. Each shaving was placed in a bowl of warm water to straighten it out. After a few minutes, each was lifted and laid on to its own glass microscope slide. When every block had been sliced in this way, the slides were placed in a basket and automatically dipped in and out of more than twenty dyes. Each dye selectively binds to a different kind of bodily cell: red blood cells become orangey-red, for instance; white blood cell nuclei are a turquoise hue; and cancer cell nuclei stain dark blue and ugly.

When Dad's slides were dry, they were mounted on to a

piece of cardboard, and most were mauve. Through a micro-scope, the samples bore little resemblance to those of healthy skin or bone, in which each cell tends to be of similar size and shape to its neighbours, each positioned in an orderly grid, like bricks in a wall or marbles in some kind of container. His cells were chaotic: some were much larger than others, and some seemed to be sprouting nodules around what had once been their smooth peripheries. Nor were they stacked with any order: in some parts of the tumour they seemed to be bunched up closely; in other parts there seemed to be gaps between the cells. To the trained eye of the pathologist, these holes indicated that the antecedents of these cells had once probably existed in a gland.

Yet there wasn't a gland in the immediate vicinity of the tumour, so Dad's cancer had not begun its life in his neck. Rather it had been created somewhere else entirely, perhaps in a gland in the stomach, or in the prostate. The tumour had probably grown there for years, encroaching on the immediate neighbourhood, until a malignant cell had floated into the bloodstream. Circulating around the body, this cell had alighted in a bone in Dad's neck, where there was a very plentiful blood supply. There it had grown into a metastasis, a secondary tumour.

§◑

From his student days Virchow had understood that scientific medicine was a battle of ideas, and in order to participate he became something of a pulpit preacher and polemicist. He often boasted to his father that these publications and public events were intended to advance his career. Indeed, the critique of Rokitansky won him the post of director of the morgue at the age of just 25, little more than a year after Marie Straide's autopsy. But the rhetoric was also aimed at changing doctors' practices and beliefs. To this end, some months after his promotion, in April 1847, he launched a journal called *Archiv für Pathologie und Medizin*. The first editorial stated that 'true science possesses the ability to act', which encapsulated his view that cold laboratory work was ineffective if it didn't affect human lives.

While Virchow laboured in the laboratory, the citizens of Berlin were gathering in beer gardens and outside the palace gates, demanding that their head of state, King Frederick William of Prussia, introduce parliamentary elections, a constitution and the freedom of the press. 'A spectre is haunting Europe,' wrote Karl Marx early in 1848, 'the spectre of Communism.' Virchow did not participate in any of these revolutionary public meetings. 'Side by side with these great events I calmly carry on my work,' Virchow wrote. At the same time, reports of a typhus epidemic in Upper Silesia in which thousands were dying was reaching Berlin. 'I have a keen desire to see it close up,' he explained. So a few days later, he persuaded the Government to allow him to tour the region and produce a scientific report. From Silesia he wrote home, reporting that a terrible famine had led to the disease, that 'the misery is endless', and worried that 'the apathy, this animal servility, is frightful'. In one town he noted that there were 3,000 orphans. Although his political masters might have expected that he would recommend a scientific solution to the problem – more doctors or more hospitals, perhaps – Virchow laid the blame on the Government for its failure to address the food shortages and on the Church for its mismanagement of the hospitals: 'one sees here quite clearly what can become of masses ground down by Catholic hierarchy and the Prussian bureaucracy'. When he returned to Berlin, ten days later, he was no longer a bystander to the revolution but felt as if medicine had carried him 'into the social sphere, there to meet some of the great problems of our time'.

On the day of his return, Friday 10 March 1848, he witnessed another series of public meetings. A few days later, citizens built barricades across various narrow streets in the city centre, the revolution having gained pace in his absence. The Government's response was robust, rapid and violent, dragoons killing several demonstrators near the royal palace, further fuelling the anger. When Virchow saw a platoon charging the crowds, wielding sabres, he realised, 'At this moment the revolution began.' That evening a running battle raged in the streets, with the royal troops firing into the crowd with cannons, pistols and shotguns. At the hospital, Virchow rushed into a colleague's office and demanded weapons, obtaining only an old gun and a rusty sabre. Guarding one of the outlying barricades, his role was 'relatively insignificant' because of the pistol's meagre range. Although he had dedicated his professional career to saving lives, he now justified taking another's on the grounds that he was defending the people from the soldiers. There was a ceasefire at 4 a.m., after which Virchow returned to the Charité where he found eleven dead civilians ready for dissection and fifty-two wounded on the wards. Elsewhere there were more corpses. Yet the violence had achieved its aim: the army and aristocrats had retreated, and the King promised a reorganisation of the Government.

'The look of Berlin today, compared with what it was fourteen days ago, is truly fantastic. Everywhere life, everywhere arms, everywhere free and public speech,' Virchow wrote a few days later. 'Perhaps the most important thing in the affair is that we have now won a feeling of self-esteem, self-respect and self-confidence.' Throughout the year, Virchow dedicated himself to the cause of the revolution, publishing a news-sheet and campaigning for democracy; 'I regard it as my civic duty to place myself at the forefront of agitation.'

Despite these efforts, within a year the Prussian aristocrats had regained power in Berlin, the old order was re-established and the revolutionary ringleaders were rounded up and executed or given long prison terms. The returning Government now accused Virchow of misusing his position at the Charité to promote the revolution. With some lobbying, Virchow avoided dismissal but was forced out of the flat he occupied in the hospital grounds. So it was fortuitous that the University of Würzberg, in Northern Bavaria, offered him a professorship, but only, some local senators insisted, if he would not turn the town into a 'playground for my hitherto demonstrated radical tendencies'. With few other options, Virchow acceded.

Virchow arrived in Würzberg in November 1849, aged 28. 'Politically all is stagnation here,' he wrote to a friend. Abstaining from politics, even disavowing his previously socialist ideas, he was dejected. 'We find ourselves in a period of deep spiritual depression in which all life has retreated to the ground of purely material interests.' Instead, he devoted himself to his young family – three of his children were born during the next few years – and to his laboratory. Indifferent to his students, who complained about his irritable manner, he found that only the microscope gave him true solace.

For the next seven years, he struggled to explain how new growths were created in the body. For the most part he held on to an idea that some kinds of speck that he had observed in the blood were in fact 'free nuclei', which became the seeds of tumours. But he never found enough evidence to formulate the idea or to promote it wholeheartedly. Instead he made only incremental contributions to science, with microscopic observations about a whole variety of tumours.

Then, in 1855, at the age of 34, he published a revolutionary editorial entitled 'Cellular Pathology' in the *Archiv*, in which he described a 'pathology of the future', a series of universal laws that described how diseases developed in the body. Two bold axioms had relevance to cancer. The first was that all cells are the product of the division of other cells or 'omnis cellula e cellula' – all cells come from cells. The second was that all abnormalities of the structure of the flesh occur because of the 'degeneration, transformations, or repetitions of normal structure', meaning that a tumour arises from a malfunctioning healthy cell in an existing organ rather than from anything in the blood, lymph or any of the body's other systems.

The theory had been based on the work of Robert Remak, a pathologist in Berlin, who being Jewish had had a fitful career as he had not been allowed to apply for certain posts. The previous year, Remak had stated that tumours 'multiply by continuous division which starts with the nucleus as I observed'. The idea had come to Remak when observing how animal embryos divided, and divided again, all future generations of cells and all future nuclei arising by this mechanism. Drawing a parallel, Remak had suggested that tumours also developed without any interference from mystical particles or free nuclei in the blood. When Virchow had reviewed this theory at the time of its publication, he had neither endorsed nor disputed it, but had only stated rather neutrally that '[Remak] finally insists as before that no free nuclei exist nor any extra-cellular creation of cells'. Yet now, a year later, Virchow had published a theory that mirrored and marginally extended Remak's without any acknowledgement to its originator.

Virchow's rivalry with Remak became all the more intense a few months after the publication of his revolutionary editorial when a professorship in pathology at the Charité Hospital in Berlin fell vacant. Virchow asked various notables to intercede on his behalf, and had copies of the editorial sent to important doctors and politicians who would influence the selection, even though he knew that the other candidate for the job was Robert Remak, the uncredited progenitor of the ideas he was now promulgating as his own.

Within a few months, in April 1856, Virchow was offered the post, just eight years after he had been forced to leave Berlin.

Virchow was similarly aggressive in a dispute that had been brewing for most of the decade. A Scottish physician called John Hughes Bennett had, for years, accused Virchow of plagiarising his own discovery of leukaemia, which had been published six weeks before Virchow's report of Marie Straide's autopsy, in 1845. In a series of vitriolic letters, Virchow defended himself by claiming that only he had realised the fundamental characteristic of the disease, that the white cells were from the blood and not from pus. His tactics were justified, he explained: 'I must be excused from entering into literary warfare against revolutionary combatants whose chief weapons are detraction and attacks on character.'

In these two incidents, Virchow prefigures many a modern cancer researcher. For in the cacophony of competing ideas, modern scientists often use not only astute laboratory science and dazzling rhetoric, but also the sharp elbows of self-advancement.

Back in Berlin, the scientific capital of the world, Virchow toured lecture theatres, promoting his idea that tumour cells grow from other cells and nowhere else. In 1858, just two years after his return, he published a book called *Die Cellularpathologie (Cellular Pathology)*, which drew a new vision of the human body, '[cells] form a free state of individuals with equal rights, though not equal abilities, which persists because individuals depend on each other'. Cancer is, therefore, a selfish and singular action of some of these cells, which by duplication threaten the body's system much as revolutionaries overturn the body politic. The book went through many German editions and was soon translated into English, the second language of science. With a few additions from other scientists, it became the accepted modern model for understanding cancer.

§

About a week after Dad's operation, we were still waiting anxiously for the news from the pathology lab. Having no knowledge of the process, we didn't understand why it was taking so long. The pathologists, meanwhile, had been rigorously running through their usual procedures, which had thus far confirmed only that the lump was cancerous.

The immunohistochemistry lab was the last port of call for Dad's cells. The technicians there would identify what kind of cells were in his tumour sample, to determine whether the malignancy originated in a gland, or if he had a carcinoma in the lining of the skin, or a lymphoma (one arising in the lymph system), or anything else. The principle underlying the tests is that each cell type can be classified according to a characteristic set of proteins called antigens, which cling to the cells' exteriors like different uniforms. Each one can be identified by a different dye. When the technician looked through the microscope at Dad's dyed cells, he confirmed that they were of the type 'adenocarcinoma', meaning that they had originated in a glandular tissue. But these tests would not reveal from what sort of gland the cells had come.

Eventually, some ten days after the operation, Dad received a letter from the hospital which first described the sample that had been excised from his neck as a three-centimetre lump of 'brownish tissue containing spicules of bone'. This disordered image of Dad's body shocked me, for it seemed to say that he was falling apart. Their conclusion was that he had 'metastatic carcinoma'.

Despite our hopes, the letter contained no ultimate explanation. The most likely site of the origin of the cancer was the prostate – a gland behind the bladder whose principal function is to produce seminal fluid – as this is the commonest form of cancer to affect men. So they tested his blood for the level of a protein called prostate specific antigen (PSA), which normally circulates around the body but can appear in greater concentrations if a tumour is present; however, on a scale where four is normal and a hundred is usually a malignant prostate cancer, Dad's PSA score was just one. Perhaps there was no tumour in his prostate. Yet, as the doctors pointed out, there was a slim possibility that Dad did have prostate cancer but had a low reading on the test, a so-called 'false negative' result. As the body is so complex, there could be many reasons for this.

With this uncertainty remaining, other tests were carried out. Dad was CAT-scanned, had MRIs and a radioactive phosphorus test, but none revealed the site of the primary tumour.

§

The paradox of cancer is that it is the wonder of life turned against itself. All life, its vibrancy and diversity, emerges from the mechanism by which a lone cell becomes two. From the beginning, an embryo is an engine of cell duplication – the fertilised egg becomes two, then four, then many, until we reach adulthood and consist of about 10 million million cells. During a lifetime, there are 100 million million of these divisions, each serving a different function, ranging a spectrum from making blood in the bone marrow to healing your wounds and, every three days, replacing the entire lining of your stomach. Taste, touch, sight, smell and hearing: all are governed by the actions of your cells. They are the bricks from which your body is built; and although each cell is an independent unit, the body relies on them to come together in an orderly way.

Similarly, for cancer to begin there need be only one malignant cell that copies itself in a chaotic and uncontrollable way; with every duplication, its dangerous characteristics are passed on to its offspring and a single aberration becomes a cluster, then a lump, then a tumour. In leukaemia, too many white blood cells are produced and so overload the blood system. In breast cancer, the natural increase in cells stimulated by the female hormone oestrogen during menstruation often becomes uncontrollable.

A year after Virchow published his *Cellular Pathology*, Darwin published *The Origin of Species*, which famously outlines his theory of 'natural selection'. In fiercely competitive environments, Darwin argues, individual animals or plants that develop useful traits will survive and multiply, whereas injurious traits will be weeded out. One example he chose was that of the wolf, which preys on various animals but is hard pressed for food during the winter season. 'Under such circumstances,' he wrote, 'the swiftest and slimmest of wolves would have the best chance of surviving, and so be preserved or selected.'

Today, Darwinism dominates scientists' ideas about cancer because the body itself is an environment in which each cell is a slightly different species; tumour cells, in particular, are constantly mutating and being selected. So with every new generation there are some cells that are better attuned to commandeering the body's resources or surviving the onslaught of various bodily chemicals. Those that are the fittest are most likely to survive.

Cancer begins when a single cell evolves into an environmental niche in which it replicates faster or dies at a slower rate than the surrounding healthy cells. A single cell can also evolve further so that it is able to float off into the bloodstream and land on a distant organ. When these so-called secondary tumours begin to grow, the whole corpus is threatened, life destroying life.

Cancer's terrible genius is that it can turn the body's natural power to the purpose of destruction. Compared to most other diseases, in which bacteria or parasites take over the body, in cancer the forces of destruction are more closely entwined with the fundamental mechanisms of life. Medicine's challenge has been to disentangle these strands so as to kill the disease while leaving the patient unharmed.

⁊

Dad and the rest of the family hungered for an obvious explanation, a primary cancer that could be excised easily and swiftly. Were he to have been afflicted with AIDS, malaria or a whole host of other illnesses, the viruses, bacteria or parasites would have been evident in any sample of blood. But Dad's primary cancer could have been a ball of flesh the size of a lentil, a few million cells large. It could have been in his prostate, in his stomach, liver or anywhere else. Even with the enormous advances in imaging technologies during the last two decades, the complex scanning machines had difficulty in distinguishing this malignant tissue from healthy cells. Without cutting him open, it was nearly impossible to know where in his body there was a tumour that was spawning others.

This lack of definite knowledge made us feel all the more impotent. Until this stage of my life, I had imagined medicine to be a precise science, a discipline of order and rationality. Yet now it appeared to be more approximate, permeated with guesswork and blind hope. The wonder that I felt for Dad's surgery was replaced by a queasy nervousness. When we asked for a more specific diagnosis, all the doctors could do was to shrug and say that when Dad had recovered sufficiently, he should undergo a course of radiation.

Radiation:
Marie Curie's new light

AFTER TEN DAYS IN HOSPITAL, Dad was discharged. At home, he slept on a bed made up in the downstairs room that served as his library. Despite the rigid plastic collar that surrounded his neck, he was able to manoeuvre himself in and out of bed. The operation seemed to have been a success.

Everything had changed, though. With Dad tired, the talking stopped earlier than it had done in previous years. He took a rainbow collection of pills, brushed his teeth at the kitchen sink (he did not have the heart for the stairs) and headed to bed. He needed assistance to ready his bedside table, which had become his command centre against nightly insomnia and pain: the radio, painkillers, a glass of water, books and walking sticks, all arranged in such a way so as not to destroy the order should he grab them in a hurry late at night. Unable now to touch his toes, he needed help in unbuckling his sandals; and his way of lying down, he joked, came from carefully studying the mechanics of his predicament. With a deft push, he would swing his legs on to the bed using the weight of his torso as a lever. There were times when this movement would induce pain, and he would ask for an adjustment of pillows or some help in shifting his body a little. When I visited, I was now the last to go to bed, and I switched off the lights.

⚜

There was a time when darkness pervaded the world, and when even the grandest of salons and the smartest of consulting rooms flickered in candle and gas lighting. Then, in the 1880s, the American inventor Thomas Edison installed an electricity generator on the Lower East Side of Manhattan and patented a mass-producible modern light bulb. Soon streets and railway stations, then surgeries and hospitals, were bathed in the light of luxury.

On 8 November 1895, a reclusive scientist called Wilhelm Röntgen in Würzberg, Bavaria, was experimenting with a three-foot-long sealed glass tube from which the air had been evacuated. Two thin wires passed through the glass and were attached to two metal plates at either end of the tube. Röntgen attached the wires to the power supply, and out of the corner of his eye he saw a sparkle of light in the darkened laboratory, apparently originating from a pile of phosphorescent crystals accidentally left on a workbench. As there was no other source of energy in the room, he realised that the phosphorescent crystals must have been sparked into emitting light by rays that were emanating from the vacuum tube. On further investigation, he discovered that although the rays were invisible to the naked eye, they shared some of the properties of light, such as travelling in a straight line. Using the phosphorescent crystals as a detector, he also discovered that the rays passed through paper but not lead. When he brought a piece of unexposed photographic paper near to the vacuum tube, the rays also created a dark cloud upon it, as if it had been left in the sunlight.

A few weeks later, he brought his wife to the laboratory. Placing her hand above a photographic plate, he bathed it in the rays for fifteen minutes. When developed, the print showed her hand as a naked skeleton with just the shadow of her flesh, her wedding ring clearly visible on one bony finger. Not knowing what to name the rays, Röntgen simply reported them as X-rays. In the following weeks, stories of his discovery, accompanied by engravings of the image of his wife's hand, were carried in newspapers all over the world.

Mystical yet modern, elusive yet scientific, X-rays captured the public imagination: jokes circulated about the need for X-ray-proof underwear, theatres produced plays with the rays as the theme; and they were demonstrated at exhibitions, where visitors were invited to stand in front of phosphorescent screens, in order to reveal the movement of their skeletons. The images' sepulchral ghoulishness was as profoundly affecting in its day as the first images of Earth from space later in the twentieth century. 'The phenomenon itself is sufficient to give us a glimpse into a new world,' the French newspaper *L'Illustration* commented, seeing the X-rays as harbingers of modernity. At the same time, these intangible products of a scientific wizardry seemed almost magical. To some, they were thought to be a dangerous meddling in the affairs of God, a premonition of death.

In medicine, X-rays were quickly used for easy diagnosis, to discover a pocket-knife lodged in the spine of a young man, for instance, or to map the fractures of limbs. They were discovered just as Victorian advances in medicine and public health, such as clean water, widespread smallpox vaccinations and better nutrition, had begun to extend life; for the first time, around 1900, the average lifespan exceeded forty years in many western countries. With the discovery of germs, safer surgery and now X-rays, faith in medicine was reaching such heights that the playwright George Bernard Shaw satirised the public's blind acceptance of the advice of avaricious practitioners in his play *The Doctor's Dilemma*. His preface helpfully reminded the audience, 'Do not try to live forever. You will not succeed.'

By contrast, by the turn of the twentieth century the incidence of cancer in America and Europe had more than tripled during the previous sixty years, and it was now the eighth leading cause of death in the United States. As there was no consensus to explain this rise, many speculated that air pollution, changes in diet, a sedentary lifestyle and over-crowded cities were to blame, almost as if cancer were a tax on civilisation. While other epidemics, such as diphtheria and scarlet fever, created greater public hysteria, cancer was becoming more of a threat; more specialised hospitals were being opened, the first cancer charities campaigned for funds, and writers described the disease. 'Cancer the Crab lies so still that you might think he was asleep if you did not see the ceaseless play and the winnowing motion of the feathery branches round his mouth,' wrote Rudyard Kipling in 1893. 'The movement never ceases. It is like the eating of a smothering fire into rotten timber in that it is noiseless and without haste.'

Within a year of the discovery of X-rays, more than 1,000 scientific papers had been published about all aspects of this 'new kind of ray'. A few years later, physicists learnt that X-rays contained the energy released when accelerated electrons hit the metal plates in the vacuum tubes.

The dangerous side effects of the rays were also soon observed. The demonstrator of an X-ray tube at a London Empire Exhibition found, for instance, that after six weeks his hands were blistering as if severely burnt. The rays' ability to burn skin was also used by doctors to treat skin rashes, ringworm and excessive hairiness. Although they understood very little about the power or behaviour of the rays, they also tried harnessing them against skin and breast cancer. Mostly amateurish, these first procedures owed more to the burlesque of a few quacks and the vision of entrepreneurs than to the practice of science.

Within a couple of years of their discovery, however, doctors had begun to rigorously experiment with the rays in treating tumours on the body's surface. Pictures of deformed, bloody cancerous boils on the necks, cheeks and heads of patients that had been transformed by X-rays into smooth, soft skin were disseminated in journals, and doctors also began to take on more challenging cases.

In November 1908, for instance, a 16-year-old girl (whose name was not included in the case report) was admitted to a Parisian hospital, having suffered from headaches, dizziness, nausea and degenerating eyesight for the previous four years; she had a squint in her right eye, one pupil did not react to brightness and she could not distinguish clearly the shapes of objects. Having stood her in front of an X-ray tube, her doctors pressed a fluoroscope, which was like a pair of binoculars attached to a small phosphorescent detection screen, to her chest. As they focused its lenses, they could see her skeleton on the screen, an image like a modern photographic X-ray. They also saw that her skull was slightly deformed, which indicated that the pituitary gland – located in the head at the base of the skull – was enlarged by a tumour that had already damaged her vision by pressing on her ocular nerve. They feared that if it continued to expand it might 'violently invade' her head. And, as the pituitary provides many of the hormones involved in growth, they also feared that her bones would gigantically extend and that her reproductive organs would not develop.

Although her doctors were ready to surgically remove the tumour, they entrusted her to a doctor called Antoine Béclère, who was Paris's leading practitioner of medical radiation. If his treatment proved ineffective, they reasoned, they could always proceed with surgery at some later date. The first session of radiation treatment took place on Saturday 5 December 1908. Béclère manoeuvred the X-ray tube – something like an oversized light bulb supported by a heavy stand – into a position twenty centimetres from her right temple, then placed a one-millimetre-thick aluminium plate between her body and the tube to act as a filter of the most scorching rays. Béclère stepped back, and clicked the switch. The mains power was more constant than the cyclist whom he had previously employed as a human dynamo, although patients still witnessed theatrical displays of sparks as the electrical systems fired up. After ten minutes, Béclère switched the machine off. Then he repeated the procedure in four more positions – above the left temple, beneath the nose and under each ear – reckoning that the pituitary gland was a little more than eight centimetres beneath the skin in each.

As the X-rays entered the flesh, they disproportionately damaged any cells that were quickly dividing, in particular, her cancer cells. Thus the numbers of cells in the tumour declined, while the surrounding tissue was left comparatively intact.

Within twenty-four hours, the girl's headaches began to diminish in both intensity and frequency. She returned for another session the following week, after which she found that her headaches ceased completely. For two months, she returned each week for another X-ray treatment. Within fifteen days, she could distinguish the numbers on the beds opposite her on the ward, as the tumour began to ease its pressure on her ocular nerve. After thirty-eight days, her eyesight was such that she wrote to her parents, 'You can see that I see much better because I can follow the lines of the paper much better. Tomorrow I get myself radiated again. That makes six or seven times. Let's hope that I will get much better.' Eight weeks after beginning the treatment, Béclère presented the case to his colleagues, declaring the method had been successful, the tumour had almost entirely disappeared, the girl was healthy and remained so.

❦

In the months after his operation, as spring turned to summer, Dad began to stretch the boundaries of his life. First he began to walk around the house, then he began climbing the stairs. Desperate to regain his mobility, he walked around the block twice a day. A month after his operation, he felt fit enough to meet his friends in the university bar. A few weeks later, he attended a gallery opening wearing a starched ruff – made by a friend who had once been a theatrical costumier – in order to hide the unsightly plastic collar that still supported his head. Dressing like a sixteenth-century gentleman generated the attention he loved. Six weeks after his operation, he began to take the plastic collar off when showering.

One Sunday, eight weeks after his operation, as we were just completing a family lunch in the garden, he disappeared into the house. After fifteen minutes, he returned and stood by the doorway, blinking into the afternoon sun. One by one each of us turned and looked in quiet admiration: his plastic collar was off, his purple shirt contrasting starkly with his pallid neck, his neck supporting his enormous head unaided. As Dad was never a man to express great emotion, I had seldom seen him so boyishly gleeful. We drank to his good health.

⁊

There is a photograph of Marie Curie taken in the first years of the twentieth century when she was in her late twenties. Around her stand the bottles, benches and notepads of a cramped and cluttered laboratory. She is dressed in a severe black dress, belted around the waist and tied at the neck; the delicate lines of her face are picked out by a gentle light. In one hand she is holding up a round-bottomed glass flask containing some unfathomable liquid, which she is staring at intently, as if she is about to make a great discovery. It is one of the many iconic images that were created in order to feed the public's insatiable desire to know about the woman who symbolised the noble endeavour of science and the hope of curing cancer.

Curie's scientific career had begun in a cold, leaky shed at the University of Paris where, in 1898, when she was just 23 years old, she and her husband had discovered a new chemical element, which she had purified from tons of an ore called pitchblende, mined from the Austrian mountains. The constant handling of the ore scarred and cracked her fingertips. It was just three years after Röntgen had discovered X-rays. When finally they isolated enough of the element to fill a tiny ampoule, they discovered that it glowed in the dark, was warm to touch and created dark shadows on photographic paper. Further investigation revealed that the element released three different sorts of rays, one of which had very similar properties to Röntgen's. Coining the term 'radioactivity' to describe this phenomenon, they called the new element 'radium'.

It was an element like almost no other. For where atoms of oxygen or carbon remained immutable, their internal atomic structure being more or less fixed and unchanged over time, radium was in a permanent state of flux, constantly expelling atoms of helium gas from within itself. During this 'cataclysm of atomic transformation', as Marie Curie once described it, the element changed itself into another called polonium, which she named after her native country, Poland. The idea that apparently inanimate matter could undergo creation and destruction revolutionised scientific thinking about the fundamental structure of atoms. 'Philosophers had only to begin their philosophy all over again and physicists their physics,' wrote Curie's daughter.

Because of the significance of Curie's discoveries, she won two Nobel Prizes: the first with her husband for physics in 1903; the second for chemistry in 1911, after he had died.

Both Marie and Pierre Curie quickly realised that radium also produced red spots, then lesions, on their skin. Like Röntgen's rays, radium therefore held out the promise of a cure for cancer. But as it released rays millions of times more powerful and could be soaked into catgut and threaded through tumours, placing the source of the radiation exactly next to the cancerous cells, the excitement was all the more intense. Certainly for cancer of the cervix and of the uterus it did prove very efficient, although the purification process was so arduous it was enormously costly to purchase.

Radium soon developed a reputation across the world as a kind of panacea – in spite of the small number of successful cases, which involved only specific parts of the body – so much so that health tonics such as 'Radium Revitalizer Water', which contained only minuscule quantities of the element, were popular, being drunk daily by at least one American president. One medical journal even suggested that it would be the 'Aladdin's Lamp to medical science'. As Marie Curie hopefully put it, 'one of the most terrible scourges, cancer, is yielding more and more to increasingly refined applications of radium, which is coming to complement or to replace surgical skills'.

Because Curie's discoveries ranged from physics to medicine, she became one of the first global celebrities in the new age of mass media. Journalists avidly chronicled each episode in her life: her husband's death in a road accident, then her affair with a married man, and the help she brought to the soldiers of the First World War, by driving X-ray machines around the battlefield of the Somme. Yet the demands of being such a public figure irritated Curie because they impinged on her time in the laboratory. After one encounter with a journalist she said, 'I feel myself invaded by a kind of stupor.' At the same time, she had always used the publicity to secure her professional positions and continued funding. As a result, she continued to receive journalists reluctantly on Thursdays and Fridays to discuss 'scientific matters' only.

When Marie Meloney, the editor of the American woman's magazine *Everybody's*, arrived at Curie's Paris laboratory in May 1920, she waited a few minutes in the small bare ante-room. Both serious and populist, her magazine featured romantic stories and dress patterns alongside articles asking 'What it means to be an American', and Meloney counted even the taciturn American Vice-President Calvin Coolidge as a close friend as well as numerous editors, politicians and writers. When Curie's door opened, Meloney later wrote, 'I saw a pale, timid little woman in a black cotton dress, with the saddest face I have ever looked upon. Her kind, patient beautiful face had the detached expression of a scholar.'

Almost as soon as they had sat down together, according to Meloney's account, Marie Curie complained that her laboratory lacked sufficient quantities of radium to continue her important work. For though there were fifty grams (almost a couple of ounces) of radium in laboratories across America, Curie explained, only a single gram existed in her institute in Paris. As 'Missy' Meloney looked around Curie's sparse lab, with its plain desk and seeming lack of equipment, she compared it to Thomas Edison's well-equipped laboratory in New Jersey, which she had recently visited to interview the inventor. Meloney later wrote that it was unfair that Curie 'had contributed to the progress of science and the relief of human suffering. And yet, in the prime of her life she was without tools which would enable her to make further contribution of her genius.'

So, on returning to America, late in the summer of 1920, Meloney set out to raise $100,000 in order to buy one gram of radium for Curie. To this end, she persuaded a group of powerful men and women, including the president of the American Medical Association and John D. Rockefeller, to join various committees to guide and give gravitas to her effort. Having convinced Curie, who hated travelling, that she should come to America to receive the present, Meloney toured newspaper offices, inspiring a campaign of hagiographic profiles and pleas for donations which culminated in the April 1921 edition of *The Delineator*, another women's magazine of which she had recently become the editor. With its editorial headline 'THAT MILLIONS WILL NOT DIE', the issue was almost entirely devoted to Curie, ending with the words, 'And life is passing and the great Curie is getting older, and the world is losing, God alone knows what great secret. And millions are dying of cancer every year.'

Curie's penury was one of Meloney's central themes in her fund-raising campaign, and she enthusiastically retold the tales of Curie's hardship during the discovery of radium. In fact, Curie's Radium Institute had been specifically built for her, to her exacting specifications, one building for the study of pure science and one for its medical applications, and had been financed mostly by philanthropic endowments; her salary was also supplemented by a special pension provided by the French Government. And even though Curie seemingly cared little for material things, she had bought several holiday homes around France, her favourite being in Cavalaire on the Riviera.

Despite her comparative prosperity, Curie was not going to refuse the generous offer of yet more help. But in the midst of this preparation, Curie became concerned that Meloney had referred to both a gram and a grain of radium in various letters. 'Marie Curie asks if one grain or one gram,' a friend of Curie's cabled. 'Grain insufficient to justify absence from work here, being one fifteenth of gram.' Meloney promised one gram, assuaging Curie who now asked whether the gift was for the University of Paris or for herself. Once again Meloney replied, 'The gram of radium is for you, for your own personal use and to be disposed of by you for use after your death.' At the same time, Meloney brokered her end of the deal by securing the first interview with Curie about the gift.

After a gala celebratory ball in her honour in Paris on 27 April 1921, Marie Curie boarded the SS *Olympic*. As it docked, two weeks later, in New York, the marching bands struck up *Le Marseillaise* and the crowds of thousands – including battalions of girl scouts and Polish women's groups – waved red and white roses. Marie Curie was sick, though, and remained below decks in the ship's best suite. When more than forty photographers and hordes of reporters, dressed in dark jackets and fedoras, rushed up the gangplank, she reluctantly gave an impromptu press conference from a large, high-backed chair on deck. Sitting implacably in her black dress, her hands entwined on her lap, she quietly responded to their questions, her daughters and Meloney standing behind her. Journalists jostled; flashbulbs popped; photographers shouted for attention. The melee marked the high point of Curie's fame, inspired by the promise of bloodless medicine.

The day after the SS *Olympic* arrived, newspapers across America ran stories about her; the *New York Times* declared, 'MME. CURIE PLANS TO END ALL CANCERS'. Never before had a scientist been so lionised for the mass audience, nor had so much been promised about the imminence of a cure for cancer. Radiation as the perfect mechanical response resonated with the ideas of the machine age: it seemed as if man was finally conquering nature, and that speed and technology were improving human life. Artists, architects and writers were passionate about the future possibilities of mechanisation, of which medical radiation was just one aspect.

The flaw was that Marie Curie's work had almost nothing to do with the treatment of cancer. True, she had discovered radium which was effective in treating uterine and cervical cancers. But she was not a physician experimenting with patients: she worked as a scientist investigating the properties of radioactive chemicals, and her insights had no relevance whatsoever in the clinic. The most concrete contribution she had made to medical practice had been to advocate a universal unit to measure the intensity of X-rays, which, in turn, meant that dosages to patients could be standardised. Even as she arrived in New York, although radium therapy for cancer was enthusiastically practised in Europe, American doctors were more cautious; the medical journals, which had once been full of radium therapy reports, now concentrated on the cheaper and more available X-rays. The public seemed to have little inkling of this change of heart. But when a reporter on the deck of the *Olympic* suggested that medical opinion was divided, Curie rebuked him: 'Nevertheless there can be positive cures when properly applied. Those who have failed, do not understand the method.'

During the following six and a half weeks, Curie was taken around America from gala balls and degree ceremonies, to university laboratories and the radium factories in Pittsburgh. In this publicity pageant, Curie had to play her part. When it was discovered that she did not own a mortar board and gown for the countless honorary degree ceremonies, Meloney sent for a tailor. Nonetheless, Curie could barely conceal her boredom. 'Shy, weary and disinterested,' lamented the *Kansas City Post*. The culmination of the trip was a reception in the White House, where President Warren Harding presented Curie with a key to a green leather case containing an hourglass inscribed with the 'Symbol and Volume of One Gram of radium'. The actual radium was still being safely kept in a factory until her departure. 'This little phial of radium,' Harding said, '[I am] confident that in your possession it will be the means to unveil the fascinating secrets of nature, to widen the field of useful knowledge, to alleviate suffering among the children of man.'

But Curie's health was declining. Her hand was in a sling, hurt by too much handshaking. As the trip progressed, she became increasingly ill and exhausted, so that she had to curtail her engagements and send her daughters instead to collect her honorary degrees. She privately acknowledged that her bouts of dizziness, drops in blood pressure and anaemia were because of 'my work with radium, especially during the war', admitting that 'it has so damaged my health as to make it impossible for me to see the laboratories and colleges in which I have a genuine interest'. Yet when her frailty was noted in the press, many reasons for it were given, from 'small talk' being too much of a burden to exhaustion from twenty years in the laboratory. Even some of the doctors who witnessed her decline refused to link her illness to radiation. 'There is no case on record of anyone being injured in health by radium,' insisted Dr E. H. Rogers, who had examined Curie, to the *New York Times*.

As her daughters attempted to disguise some of Curie's woes, more trips were cancelled. By the end of June, the family were back aboard the *Olympic*, Europe bound. In the purser's safe was the coveted gram of radium – sealed in a lead pot, which had been placed in a wooden box.

❧

Three months after his operation, the slow upward trajectory of my father's recovery seemed to stall. Tired and annoyed, he became frustrated that the wonder of health seemed, once again, to be slipping away. He was not sleeping well, and was also losing the strength in his arms. If I held up my hands and asked him to push against me, something he would easily have been able to do just a few weeks before, he could muster no force at all. I felt that in his depression he was losing the will to recover. I berated him for not trying to stand more often or to push harder, but he would just laugh at me. A materialist shouldn't believe so much in mind over matter, he'd say. Once, while shopping, I wanted him to carry something in the belief that the weight on his arms might prevent them from atrophying. Whether or not this was true, it would be a symbol of his fight. So I gave him a shopping bag. When he winced and dropped it, I realised that he was trying but simply could not manage it. I progressively emptied the contents of his bag into mine. In the end, all he could cope with was a single bag of pasta. As we walked home, I hoped at least this small muscular exercise might be doing him some good.

A week after he had begun to lose power in his arms,

he returned to hospital for another series of scans, which seemed to suggest that some stray cells of his tumour remained in his neck. As these had continued to replicate, they had put pressure on the nerves that ran across his back into his arms.

&

On her return to Paris, in 1921, Marie Curie continued to investigate the basic properties of atoms using radium. At the same time, the head of the medical section of her institute, a doctor called Claudius Regaud, was embarking on a series of experiments that would fundamentally change how X-rays were given to patients. Experimenting on the testes of rams, whose cells he imagined might replicate rather like a tumour's, he discovered that many small bursts of radiation, given over some days, were more likely to make them infertile than a single equivalently powered blast. As a result, Regaud created a rationale for 'fractionation', in which cancer patients are given many smaller doses rather than a single large dose, which as well as being more effective also minimises skin burns and the more general side effects of tiredness and lethargy – a method still used today.

The reason fractionation works is that there are certain stages of a cell's life-cycle when it is more endangered by radiation. In the case of most cells, radiation will fatally damage them at the moment of division, but not during the process when the chromosomes are being duplicated that precedes it. This means that in any tumour there are some cells which are killed by a particular burst of radiation, while others survive. Those that endure continue to live, and replicate at varying speeds. So twenty-four hours after the first dose of radiation, another group of cells will be vulnerable to X-rays. Repeating daily doses whittles away at the tumour.

❧

The problem with Dad's arms had arisen because his neck had needed time to heal. A course of radiation would have killed not only the remaining cancer cells but also those normal fast-growing cells necessary to repair his wounds. In properly prioritising Dad's neck, the doctors had nonetheless given the cancer the opportunity to return in the three months since his operation.

Now that Dad could hold up his head, however, radiation therapy could be attempted and every day Dad walked a mile to the hospital. The machines were much more powerful, and more accurate, than those of Marie Curie's day. He lay down on his front, his head supported by pillows. The machine whirred into its position and delivered the dose. A few minutes later, he was told he could go. For ten days he returned every day, receiving quite a large dose but suffering very few side effects.

After a week, the tumour apparently no longer pressed against his arm nerves, and Dad began to feel his muscles again. After ten days, as the cancer disappeared somewhat, he slowly regained the use of his arms. For the first time since his operation, he was now able to sleep through the night without being woken by pain.

❧

In 1921, some months after Curie had left America, Amelia Maggia, a 22-year-old woman from Orange, New Jersey, became so weak and tired she had to quit her job. A few streets away, a 20-year-old, Irene Rudolph, began to suffer from a sore throat and a swollen face, then aching teeth and gums. Weeks later, another local woman, 20-year-old Hazel Vincent, began to experience pains in her teeth. After her dentist pulled a tooth, the scar never healed. By the spring of 1922, Amelia Maggia's bones had deteriorated so much that her dentist was able to lift her entire lower jawbone from her mouth when he was trying to treat her teeth. A few months later, she died. At first these seemed to be isolated incidents in this town, which was teeming with first-generation Italian and Irish immigrants, but others soon began to fall ill: Marguerite Carlough, Katherine Schaub, Genevieve and Josephine Smith, and Helen Quinlan. When Irene Rudolph's cheek swelled up and her mouth began to hurt, her dentist removed a tooth but the socket never healed. She died in 1923, from 'a most terrible and mysterious illness', according to her cousin.

The afflicted convened an informal meeting in January 1924, at the office of one of their dentists. As they talked, it became clear that all had worked at the dial-painting studio of the US Radium Corporation. The company owned uranium mines on the Colorado plateau, using its Orange workshop to produce luminous watch faces, which were very fashionable at the time; in 1919 alone, more than 2 million watches were produced by US Radium and their competitors. The girls enjoyed working in the light and airy workshop, where they were allowed to chatter and laugh as they mixed the paint, dipped their brushes and licked them to keep them pointed. They also made mischief with the luminous paint by decorating their fingernails and eyelids – and one girl had even surprised her date with a Cheshire Cat grin by painting her teeth. Even when they returned home, their clothes still gave off a gentle light in the darkness of their bedrooms. Nobody had imagined that the small doses of radium in the paint, about 1 part per 30,000, could be, in any way, harmful. After all, large numbers of people were still regularly drinking Radium Revitalizer Water, which contained minuscule quantities of the element and was sold everywhere.

When the vice-president of the company was told that dentists were making claims that 'work in our application department is hazardous and has caused injury and poor health', he wrote to the insurance company, saying, 'We do not recognize that there is such a hazard to the occupation.' Most other experts would have agreed with this opinion, for although it was widely acknowledged that large doses of radium damaged the body's cells, few people realised that the tiny quantities in paint could cause any harm.

In March 1925, with four dial painters already dead, Marguerite Carlough filed a suit against US Radium, claiming damages of $75,000, four years after falling ill. She had started dial painting at the age of 18 and had worked in the studio for four years. This first court case was reported by the newspapers; as the dangers of radium crept into the public consciousness, the company settled out of court for $9,000. In December, at the age of 24, Carlough died of anaemia, pneumonia and, as her niece described, 'a horrible jaw problem'.

That year, Missy Meloney informed Marie Curie of the dial workers' deaths. Like many others at the time, Marie Curie held somewhat contradictory views about the dangers of radiation. On the trip to America she had admitted that her own scarred fingertips and anaemia had been caused by the large doses she had received in the early years, or when she was wheeling X-ray machines around during the First World War. At other times she was more doubtful: 'Perhaps radium has something to do with these troubles, but it cannot be confirmed with any certainty.' And although many of her co-workers suffered from all kinds of similar diseases, she was often unwilling, except in the most obvious cases, to make a connection with radiation. Particularly, she did not think that prolonged exposure created permanent damage that fresh air could not undo. When her daughter, who also worked with radium, saw her blood count become abnormal in 1927, Marie wrote to her brother, 'She will be leaving soon for two weeks of winter sports and hopes that this stay in the mountains will be good for her anaemia.'

In New Jersey, month by month, girl after girl succumbed. By 1927, thirteen had died from the so-called 'radiation necrosis'. One of those still alive was a 28-year-old woman called Grace Fryer, who had been suffering from pains in her bones for four years and had worked at US Radium some years before. But even sympathetic doctors were worried about the unwarranted publicity. 'If radium has unknown dangers, it might seriously injure the therapeutic use of radium,' said Charles Norris, the chief medical examiner of New York. Eventually, Fryer persuaded a young attorney called Raymond Berry, who had only recently graduated from Harvard, to take on her case on a contingency basis.

In May 1927, he filed the first case for Grace Fryer in the New Jersey Supreme Court. Four other women, Edna Hussman, Katherine Schaub and sisters Quinta McDonald and Albina Larice quickly joined the lawsuit, each asking for $250,000 in compensation for medical expenses and pain. By the time the case eventually arrived in the courtroom, in January 1928, the health of all five women had deteriorated. Grace Fryer, in particular, was declining rapidly: she had lost all of her teeth, she could not sit up without a back brace, and she had to be wheeled to the witness stand. None of the five victims, whom the press called the 'Radium Girls', was able to raise their hand to swear the oath. 'FIVE WOMEN SMILE, FEARING DEATH, IN RADIUM CASE' was the headline in the *Newark Ledger* on 18 January: 'When pretty Grace Fryer took the witness stand, she said her health had been good until after she had been employed at the radium plant.'

By April of that year, the women were not physically able to attend the second court hearing. Even though Berry objected strenuously to an adjournment, the judge set a new date in September, so that US Radium's witnesses would be able to attend. In response, the press, led by Walter Lippmann, the editor of the *New York World*, was outraged. The delay, he wrote in an editorial, was a 'damnable travesty of justice ... If ever a case called for prompt adjudication, it is the case of five crippled women who are fighting for a few miserable dollars to ease their last few days on earth.' With the girls' deaths imminent, and the publicity damaging the company, all parties agreed to an out-of-court settlement of $15,000 and further necessary medical expenses for each girl.

The flurry of publicity revealed a dark side to the dream of modernity that had been sparked thirty years before. That technology could be dangerous became a significant motif of the culture of the time. In the film *The Invisible Ray* (1936), Boris Karloff played a demented scientist bent on an evil rampage after being poisoned by radiation. And in Aldous Huxley's *Brave New World* (1932), one of the characters expresses his rejection of the utopian world state by demanding that alongside the right to be unhappy, he ought to have the right to contract cancer.

With the deaths of the girls, therefore, radiation became not only a modern symbol for healing but also for destruction. And as these stories had bubbled up just as mass media was being created, they foreshadowed the hyperbole created in response to both other 'cures' and other possible risks that emerged later in the century. Yet in the case of radiation, as well as many of the later stories, the distorted picture that was painted was both overly hopeful and too despairing. In fact, radiation was not a threat to the general population, although of course there were dangers – for pregnant women, for instance, or for children when X-rays were used for shoe-fitting. And these dangers were slowly erased from human experience. But nor was it a panacea against the disease. Nonetheless, during the 1920s and 1930s, medicine was incrementally and painstakingly advancing, and radiation was extending lives.

By the mid 1930s, millions of volts, rather than tens of thousands, were driving the X-ray tubes. With beams able to penetrate deeper into the body, it was possible to treat the stomach, for instance, rather than only the neck, breast and skin. In tandem, doctors began to learn how to more finely control the beams, so that they would accurately target the tumour rather than the surrounding healthy flesh. By the late

1930s, radiation therapy jostled with surgery as the first line of treatment against many cancers. Many of the machines that now treat patients are direct descendants of those early creations; but they are now more powerful, and are helped by computers to map exactly the position of the tumour.

In 1931, twenty-three years after Antoine Béclère irradiated that unnamed 16-year-old girl who had been admitted to the Parisian hospital with deteriorating eyesight, she wrote to him, because she had just given birth to a healthy child.

In July 1934, Marie Curie died of a pneumonia, a complication of aplastic anaemia caused by radiation.

Although the element radium itself has been superseded in cancer medicine, the principle of placing radioactive material near cancers remains.

❧

As Dad returned to health after his radiation therapy, about five months after his first diagnosis, I found that my emotions were swinging from hope to despair. There were times when it was as if thoughts of his disease had been banished from his mind, when the experience of those slow summer days, with Dad pouring drinks and cooking food, had erased the memories of the crisis that had occurred just a few months before. But fear was never far away. After a few days of optimism, I began to worry that this was no more than a temporary pause before a further decline. Nervously, I monitored the way he now used the cutlery for signs of weakness; when he went for walks, I would hang back, studying the way he held his shoulders.

Slowly, as the days turned to weeks and then months and he remained healthy, my family and I pushed worry from our minds, at least momentarily, as if we needed a respite from the burden. Freed from the day-to-day concern, we began to think more broadly about Dad's disease, and ask: what might have caused it?

Causes:
is civilisation the problem?

WHEN I WAS 14, Dad gave me a book by Rachel Carson called *Silent Spring*. Dad told me that when he first read the book, as a series of long articles in the *New Yorker* in 1962, Carson's vision – of how modern chemicals, and in particular the insecticide DDT, were poisoning rivers, polluting the air and destroying wildlife – had transformed his world view. 'A grim spectre has already silenced the spring in countless towns in America,' she states.

Twenty years later, when Dad and I first began to talk about the history of cancer, I picked up the book. It begins with 'A Fable for Tomorrow': a futurological sketch of a town at 'the heart of America' where a blight has stopped the birds from singing. She also describes the devastating effects of chemicals on the population: 'Everywhere was a shadow of death. The farmers spoke of much illness among their families. In the town the doctors had become more and more puzzled by new kinds of sickness appearing among their patients.'

The rest of the book documents how the misuse of pesticides, herbicides and other synthetic chemicals was already creating this nightmare vision. With chapter headings such as 'Elixirs of Death', 'Needless Havoc' and 'Rivers of Death' there is little ambiguity in Carson's anger and passion: 'For the first time in the history of the world, every human being is now subjected to contact with dangerous chemicals, from the moment of conception until death.'

Her contribution to our understanding of cancer is in a chapter entitled 'One in Every Four', which refers to rates of incidence of the disease; this has since increased to one in every three. 'With the dawn of the industrial era the world became a place of continuous ever-accelerating change. Instead of the natural environment there was rapidly substituted an artificial one composed of new chemical and physical agents, many of them possessing powerful capacities for inducing biologic change,' wrote Carson. These dangerous chemicals 'have entered the environment of everyone – even of children as yet unborn. It is hardly surprising, therefore, that we are now aware of an alarming increase of malignant disease.'

Silent Spring was profoundly influential as the foundation of the environmental movement. As well as selling hundreds of thousands of copies in both America and Europe, it achieved some policy changes. The establishment of the US Government's Environmental Protection Agency in 1970 and the banning in America of the pesticide DDT in 1974 were in part due to this book.

The idea that the rising incidence of cancer is due to the increased amounts of pesticides, fertilisers, food colouring and such like released into the air, rivers and food chain by modern industry has also remained pervasive. Today, newspapers regularly run features about industrial toxins that lurk beneath our skins, threatening cancer with every turn; and the organic food industry is on the rise in part because of a fear that pesticides are ruining our health.

Yet even as Rachel Carson was promoting these ideas about cancer, few scientists believed them to be true. Mainstream cancer institutions and many doctors still remain opposed to them. For although Carson presents her polemic as timeless and universal, a critique of modern life for all time, her ideas were very much rooted in a series of very specific concerns of her day. The environmental theory of cancer, in particular, had been created in response to a cancer epidemic that was sweeping the industrial world. It was authored, for the most part, by Wilhelm Hueper, a German immigrant to America whose research Carson used in writing *Silent Spring*. As the director of the Environmental Health Section of the US Government's National Cancer Institute, in Bethesda, Maryland, Hueper was regarded by Carson as the 'foremost authority on environmental cancer', and he is referred to repeatedly throughout her book. And it is his concerns, therefore, which were forged in the 1930s, that continue to be of influence.

&.

Wilhelm Hueper was born in Germany in 1894. Having fought in the First World War, he trained to be a doctor, and then travelled to America at the age of 29 because inflation was threatening his livelihood. Although he lived there for the rest of his life, he never lost his thick accent. He also retained something of an immigrant's sensibility, opposed to the existing order of the cancer establishment.

He had arrived in America at the same time as public concerns about cancer were rising; incidence was increasing at an annual rate of 2.5 per cent. With each passing year, another statistic emphasised the danger: by 1924, cancer had surpassed tuberculosis as a cause of death in America; by 1934, it had become the nation's number two killer after heart disease. Senator Matthew Neely of West Virginia captured the mood in 1929, when he described, 'a monster that is more insatiable than the guillotine, more destructive to life and health than the mightiest army that has ever marched to battle, more terrifying than any scourge that has ever threatened the existence of the human race'. In Neely's apocalyptic vision, cancer would 'depopulate the earth'.

Yet there was still no consensus on the cause of the epidemic; rather, there was a series of competing ideas of varying rationality. Some scientists claimed that the increasing rates were the remnants of the influenza epidemic of 1918, others that cancer was caused by the spread of tar on roads, the increased numbers of trout in freshwater streams, tuberculosis, the acidity of blood, viruses or the consumption of tomatoes. There was even a large body of scientific opinion that argued that rates of cancer incidence were not rising at all, but rather medicine had become better at detecting and diagnosing something that had always existed.

Even Freudian psychoanalysts contributed to the debate, by updating a Galenic idea and suggesting that people with a melancholic disposition and repressed sexuality were more susceptible to the disease. As the poet W. H. Auden put it at the time, 'Nobody knows what the cause is / Though some pretend they do / It's like some hidden assassin / Waiting to strike at you.' But amidst all the confusion about the cause, the general feeling was that cancer was linked to civilisation, that industrialisation, which had once been heralded as the creator of a new world, was now a harbinger of illness and death.

By 1930, the 35-year-old Hueper was working at the University of Pennsylvania, in a laboratory funded by Irénée du Pont, the chairman and largest shareholder of DuPont Chemicals. The company made gun-powder and produced all kinds of newfangled compounds essential to modern life: Freon, a chloro fluoro carbon (CFC) refrigerant; synthetic rubber and lacquer finishes for automobiles; as well as essential additives for gasoline and cellophane for food preservation.

That summer, Wilhelm Hueper arranged a visit to DuPont's Deepwater Chemical Works, in New Jersey, a sprawling city of brick warehouses, covering 1,500 acres.

Steam and smoke billowed from each building, and thousands of tons of poisonous effluent ran into the River Delaware. On calm days, the fumes hung in the air, irritating the throats of less-inured visitors. Observing how a range of chemicals called aromatic amines were used to produce certain dyes, such as mauve and scarlet, Hueper remembered a scientific paper that he had read when he had been translating German abstracts for the American *Archives of Pathology* a few years before. On returning to his lab, he tracked down these reports and wrote a memorandum to Irénée du Pont that explained how scientists in Germany, Switzerland and England had recently suspected aromatic amines to have caused bladder cancer in dye workers, and warned of the danger in Deepwater. Hueper received no response. Then, a few months later, Dr Ellice McDonald, the head of the laboratory and also the du Pont family's physician, passed on the message that no cancers had been discovered among the Deepwater workers.

Mainstream medical opinion was similarly sceptical of the idea that industrial chemicals could cause cancer, in exactly the same way that the risks of radium had been ignored in the dial-painting factory in Orange, New Jersey, a few years earlier. Though Sir Percival Pott from St Bartholomew's Hospital in London had drawn the link in 1775 between soot and scrotal cancer, there had since been only a small number of studies which indicated that industrial chemicals might contribute to the disease, and few of them were regarded as significant. This was, after all, a time when synthetic materials such as nylon heralded a future of iron-free leisure, and when chemicals became wonder drugs – such as one called '606', which treated syphilis and so captured the public imagination that the drug's inventor would soon be immortalised in a Hollywood film entitled *Dr Ehrlich's Magic Bullet*. Hueper's criticism was seen, therefore, as a polemic against progress.

A few months after du Pont had rejected the link between aromatic amines and bladder cancer, the company's medical director arrived without an appointment at Hueper's laboratory, late one afternoon. Dr George Gehrmann told Hueper he was distinctly alarmed, having just discovered twenty-three bladder cancer cases among hundreds of the dye workers. As the previous European reports had shown that the tumours typically arose ten to fifteen years after exposure to the chemicals, and as dye production had begun at DuPont in 1917, Hueper explained that 'a new industrial hazard of industrial origin had arrived on schedule in the United States'.

The lesson that Hueper took from this discovery was that all industrial chemicals and their by-products ought to be 'studied for their toxic and pharmacologic properties for the protection of the producers as well as the consumers'. Although Hueper suggested, soon after, that the DuPont Company establish an institute for such research, Irenée du Pont said that the Depression was 'impairing the availability of the necessary funds'.

For four years, Hueper continued his career as a laboratory pathologist. But by 1934 his relationship with Dr Ellice McDonald had soured, and he was dismissed. In the face of the Depression, he returned to his homeland with his wife. 'We decided to test our luck in Germany, where openings had become available because of the Hitler turmoil,' he wrote, sketching over the fact that these 'openings' resulted from the recent Nazi law which proscribed Jews from working for the state. At the Charité Hospital in Berlin, for example, twelve of the thirteen scientists working on cancer research had been dismissed. In preparation for his journey, Hueper wrote speculative letters of introduction to various scientists and government ministers, signing at least one of them, 'Heil Hitler!'

By the time Hueper arrived in Germany, in the late summer of 1934, Hitler had been Chancellor for only a year, but there was already an emerging political campaign against what the Nazis believed to be cultural causes of cancer. Leading the fray was a Danzig surgeon called Erwin Liek who had recently published a book entitled *The Spread, Prevention and Control of Cancer*, which stated that 'the simpler and more natural one's way of life, the rarer cancer'. Rising cancer rates were the result, he believed, primarily of bad nutrition, including the toxic effect of colourings in food and white breads. In addition, excessive smoking and drinking, the new and widespread use of arsenic pesticides and artificial fertilisers, and sexual promiscuity were causes.

However, Liek was optimistic, promising that Germans would soon practise 'cancer prevention on a large scale – for the entire people', rather than just 'care for the individual'. As he was close to the Nazi Party, and had been asked by Hitler to be the leader of the medical profession under his regime, Liek's opinions became the foundation for a wide-ranging public health campaign that developed during the Nazi period and included posters promoting healthy German bread, school-books encouraging the eating of fruit and vegetables, and regulations controlling occupational carcinogens such as asbestos.

These campaigns echoed Hitler's own beliefs; he was himself a vegetarian. Ever since he had witnessed his mother's death from breast cancer in 1907, when he was 18, he had been interested in the disease. The intensity of Hitler's fascination was particularly evident during the morning of the invasion of the Soviet Union in June 1941, when he broke off from working on his speech to talk with Joseph Goebbels about the latest results of cancer research. The month of Hueper's arrival, September 1934, Hitler had even had the Chancellery examined for 'earth rays' – some kind of radiation that the earth was supposed to emit – for fear that they might cause cancer.

Hueper's first job interview was with a certain Professor Fischer-Wasels in Frankfurt, who, much like Liek, seemed somewhat influenced by the ideas of the times, declaring that a nascent tumour was a 'new race of cells, distinct from the other cell races in the body'. Well known among scientists for showing that a scarlet dye induced tumours in the ears of rabbits, Fischer-Wasels told Hueper that such a demonstration would be impossible under the Nazis because Goering had banned all animal experiments. As there was the possibility of more restrictions, he advised Hueper to return to America. Hueper failed to find work in Frankfurt, but went for meetings in Heidelberg, Berlin, Freiburg and then on to Munich, where his application was refused by a Nazi Party representative. 'The adventure was over without yielding any hope. It had become clear that my destiny and that of my family was definitely in the United States.' As Hueper packed his steamer trunk on to the boat at Bremerhaven, he was participating in a westward migration of scientific talent; the dominance that Germany had enjoyed over world medicine for a century and more was over.

On his return to America, the DuPont company offered him work investigating the problem of bladder cancer, in their new occupational health laboratory. At first it seemed as if he had found a place which shared his interests. But after three years, the laboratory's director began to restrict the type of experiments Hueper could carry out: he was not allowed, for instance, to test the long-term effects of certain chemicals on animals – experiments which Hueper believed would be necessary to prove their latent dangers. He was also prevented from publishing some of his research, with the claim that it contained commercial secrets. Hueper was dismissed in 1937. Yet the reluctance of industry to investigate the dangers that it was producing only hardened Hueper's resolve.

In the months of searching for a new post, he dedicated himself to cataloguing every chemical that caused cancer. Travelling to medical libraries in New York and Philadelphia, he read scientific papers from the previous century that documented how such things as soot, uranium or tanning oils had damaged various groups of workers. He filed the evidence on hundreds of cards, which he piled high on his dining-room table. When he eventually found work, in 1938, at William R. Warner Pharmaceuticals, they allowed him to continue this great endeavour. The magnum opus that resulted was called *Occupational Tumors and Allied Diseases* and was eventually published in 1942. Running to almost a thousand pages, the book argued that the cancer epidemic was due to the 'rise in the modern and artificial environment'. The never-ending numbers of chemicals that humans now came into contact with – including 'dyes, mordants, explosives, plastics, fertilizers, insecticides, fungicides, solvents, rubber, resins, lacquers, pigments, paints, finishes, textile fibers, fuel and lubricants for motors and machines, refrigerants, building materials, radioactive substances, food components, drugs, toilet articles, pharmaceuticals, household supplies, and innumerable articles' – were, Hueper believed, linked to the rising incidence of cancer. However, simple precautions could, according to Hueper, curtail the epidemic.

Although Hueper's book was the first comprehensive classification of the cancerous damage caused by industrial chemicals, none of the recently emerged cancer journals carried a review. *The Lancet* in London printed a barbed attack by the most eminent researcher in the field, Sir Ernest Kennaway, entitled 'A Contribution to the Mythology of Cancer Research', which argued that Hueper had exaggerated some of the historical evidence and had reached conclusions about the effects of environmental carcinogens that were insufficiently grounded in the evidence. Hueper responded in a typically belligerent manner by accusing Kennaway of 'prejudice and perversion'. In general, the book inspired little enthusiasm, the ongoing war being more important to most doctors.

However, by 1945, Hueper's achievements began to be recognised: the editor of the *Journal of the American Medical Association* asked him, for instance, to write a number of editorials on the subject of environmental carcinogens.

In 1947, Hueper's reputation was such that when the US Government's National Cancer Institute established the Environmental Cancer Section, he was chosen to be its first director.

Shortly after Hueper's arrival at the National Cancer Institute, Dr George Gehrmann – the medical director of the DuPont company who in 1930 had discovered the twenty-three bladder cancer cases – wrote to the Federal Loyalty Commission claiming that Hueper was a Nazi, in a somewhat crude attempt to discredit a vocal critic who was a threat to the profits of the chemical industry. When the first letter failed to dent Hueper's reputation, more letters were sent suggesting he had 'communistic tendencies'. Similarly, when Hueper attempted to persuade the chemical industry to cooperate in the discovery of chemical carcinogens, DuPont refused to participate.

Even within the Government there was concern that Hueper was attempting to frustrate important industrial and scientific advances. His interest in the lung cancers of uranium mine-workers on the Colorado plateau provoked particular unease, reaching a climax in 1952, when the US Government's Atomic Energy Commission instructed him to eliminate all mentions of radiation hazards from a report. In response, Hueper publicly claimed that he was being asked to be a 'scientific liar', whereupon the Atomic Energy Commission demanded that Hueper be dismissed.

Although he just managed to retain his post, his superiors in the National Cancer Institute were finding it impossible to defend him continually. A few months later, a representative of the chromate industry wrote to the US Surgeon General complaining about Hueper. The Surgeon General's response was to prohibit him from unearthing any more information about the detrimental effects of chemicals on humans, placing him in the absurd position, as a high-ranking public health official, of no longer having contact with patients, or being able to investigate how chemicals caused cancer in man. He was only allowed to work with laboratory animals.

The wilful disregard of the problems of chemicals by both industry and government toughened Hueper's stance. Throughout the early 1950s, he gave evidence to a variety of congressional committees calling for the investigation of these chemicals. It was evidence that Rachel Carson would draw heavily upon when she was writing *Silent Spring* a decade later. Yet Wilhelm Hueper's belief that environmental chemicals could explain the cancer epidemic was facing a more powerful threat than even industry or government: an alternative theory.

❧

Four months after his operation, and a month after the radiation therapy, Dad seemed to be returning to his old self. Although he was gaining in strength, I worried about the small things, such as his insistence on drinking wine or his taking little exercise. I would quietly voice my concern that perhaps he was aggravating his disease. As he always had, he calmly dismissed my suggestions. After all, he'd say, the damage is already done. In any case, he was hungry for the tiny luxuries of living, for it was these that proved he had survived.

On one occasion, we began discussing what might have caused the disease. Then he climbed up the stairs to his office on the top floor of the house. Though the sea of papers balanced on boxes looked chaotic, he had a system. He rifled through one of his filing cabinets and pulled out an offprint of a paper from the 1950s by two epidemiologists called Richard Doll and Austin Bradford Hill. Perhaps this might be of interest, he said.

Throughout my adolescence, over the Saturday breakfast Dad read each of Richard Doll's scientific papers that appeared in Mum's weekly copy of the *British Medical Journal*.

As one of the most eminent epidemiologists of his era, Doll's papers ranged widely, each one describing the various links between certain aspects of human life, such as diet or industrial asbestos, and such epidemics as heart disease and cancer. Doll was a man, Dad often told me, with a gift for discovering the patterns of disease from the millions of pieces of information generated by studying the behaviour of thousands of individuals, a skill like being able to see the correct figure in a pointillist painting while others saw only coloured dots or imagined the wrong image entirely. As Doll's rise to prominence had begun just as Dad was beginning his own academic career in a related subject, Dad looked up to him. When Dad began to teach statistics at the University of Aberdeen in 1951, one of his favourite topics was the medical statistics that Richard Doll was pioneering at the time.

&

Doll had been born in 1912. He had trained as a doctor, but soon realised that he loved numbers more than individual patients; even as a student he had used statistics to demonstrate that one senior surgeon's chosen operation cured patients no better than no intervention whatsoever. Where Wilhelm Hueper's beliefs were rooted for the most part in the pathology of dead bodies, the symptoms of individual cases and the study of animals, Richard Doll, who was eighteen years younger, believed that the emerging field of statistics, its collation of vast numbers of results, could demonstrate as yet undiscovered truths about diseases in human populations.

At the age of 36, in 1948, he was asked by Austin Bradford Hill, then the leading medical statistician of the day, to join a research project that had been initiated by the British Government to explain why lung cancer rates had increased sixfold during the previous twenty years. A growing number of statistics now showed that it was lung cancer, which had barely existed at the beginning of the century, that was responsible for the large increase in cancer deaths, rather than there being a cancer epidemic affecting all locations in the body. At the time, there seemed to be a large number of possible causes: the production of gas by smelting coal; improved standards of diagnosis, which were identifying more cases; or the London smog, which was often of such severity that visibility dropped to just a few feet (once Doll had to ask his wife to lead the car on foot because he could not see anything). Somewhere near the bottom of the list was the smoking of cigarettes. 'If I had to put money on anything at the time I should put it on motor exhausts or possibly on the tarring of roads,' remembered Doll, who was himself a smoker. 'But cigarette smoking was such a normal thing and had been for such a long time that it was difficult to think it could be associated with any disease.'

Doll knew of one statistical study that linked smoking to cancer: a research project that had been carried out in Nazi Germany by a 25-year-old student called Franz Müller, who had, in 1939, surveyed eighty-six male lung cancer patients at a hospital in Cologne. At the time, most scientific papers were based on case studies that described the symptoms of each patient throughout the development of their disease, rather like a series of pen portraits, but Müller had attempted to analyse the group of patients as a whole. To do so he had matched each male patient to another man of a similar age who did not have lung cancer, thereby creating a so-called 'control group' whose differences and similarities could be compared with the diseased group, in a method called 'case-control'. The results were startling: lung cancer patients were six times more likely to be 'extremely heavy smokers' than those who were not. So Müller had concluded that tobacco was the 'single most important cause of rising incidence of lung cancer'.

Müller's study had coincided with a comprehensive Nazi anti-smoking drive that included restrictions on advertising, bans on smoking in post offices and trains, a children's education programme, and a poster campaign portraying the good workers who abstained. Such was the Nazi fervour against smoking that during the war Stalin, Roosevelt and Churchill were portrayed by Government propaganda as smokers, contrasting with the clean fascists, Hitler and Mussolini. When an anti-tobacco research institute opened in Jena, in Germany, in 1941, it was funded by the *Reichskanzelei*, the office of the head of state. 'Best of luck in your work to free humanity from one of its most dangerous poisons,' telegrammed the Führer for the inauguration. These measures made Nazi Germany the only country in the world that was attempting to save the majority of its citizens from cancer – while simultaneously committing genocide.

In London in the spring of 1948, little was known about the wider anti-smoking policy of the Nazis, although Müller's research paper remained publicly available. Doll remained sceptical, however, of Müller's bold conclusions, not least because they had been drawn from the experience of such a small number of patients. So Doll instructed four social workers to collect information about patients suspected of having lung cancer in twenty London hospitals, asking about their smoking habits, their occupations, their age and whether they worked with coal gas or near roads. Given that the symptoms of lung cancer were so often confused with those of diseases such as tuberculosis, Doll's task was then to confirm the diagnosis upon each patient's death or discharge. As Doll interviewed doctors and read the case notes, he soon realised that there was a striking anomaly: the smokers in the study invariably had lung cancer, while the non-smokers had usually been incorrectly diagnosed. As a consequence, even before the results had been properly analysed, Doll himself gave up smoking within a year of commencing the study.

By the beginning of 1950, Doll and Hill had 649 case histories of lung cancer patients, as well as those of a comparable number of other patients of a similar age without tumours, the 'control group'. The conclusion was that the risk of developing lung cancer was '50 times as great among those who smoke 25 or more cigarettes a day as among non-smokers'. Though the results were astonishing, the then head of the British Medical Research Council suggested that because the research had been carried out only in London there might be an error. So he advised similar research in cities throughout England before publication.

However, there were other researchers pursuing similar lines of enquiry, and in May 1950 the *Journal of the American Medical Association* published a similar study of 684 in patients Chicago, St Louis and California carried out by a young doctor called Ernst Wynder. Disappointed at having been pre-empted, Doll and Hill published their own report a few months later in the *British Medical Journal*.

Neither report had any real impact. At a time when more than two-thirds of all American and British men were smokers, it was seemingly hard to accept that this could be damaging. Sceptical scientists argued, for instance, that there was only one study worldwide which showed that cigarette smoke caused tumours in animals – and this had been carried out in Brazil, a long way from the established centres of scientific excellence. Other critics doubted that smoke could travel to every corner of the lung where tumours had been observed. To counter this, Doll went to the Hammersmith Hospital in West London, where he was to inhale radio-actively tagged smoke that would be mapped by X-ray. As the laboratory smoke was acrid and foul, Doll coughed and spluttered, failing to inhale deeply enough. Although he tried repeatedly, in the end he abandoned the experiment.

One reason that Doll and Hill had trouble convincing the world of their argument was that their statistical methods were new. Doctors were more used to deducing causes of disease after seeing bacteria or a virus in the blood or cadaver than relying on Doll and Hill's complicated numbers, which were open to wide interpretation. So although Doll and Hill had shown that lung cancer patients seemed more likely to be smokers than non-smokers, many others refused to believe that cigarettes were the *cause* of this disparity. It was similar to the classic scientific error: though a particular group of chestnut horses might, in a facile example, be faster than a comparable group of grey stallions, it would be wrong to conclude that this was because of their colour.

The weakness of the study, which Doll and Hill acknowledged, was the biases that might have been introduced unknowingly. In particular, the group under study was far from typical of the normal population, as they were in hospital already. Moreover, taking the smoking histories from those suffering from lung cancer was prone to error as patients might embroider the truth: healthy heavy smokers might be likely to underestimate their intake, while those already ill might exaggerate their past indulgence.

To overcome these biases, Richard Doll and Austin Bradford Hill invented an entirely new method of medical research: rather than looking to patterns in the past, they would track the lives, habits and deaths of a large number of men and women over the coming years, in the hope that time would demonstrate the cause of the deaths of those who admitted to being smokers at the beginning of the study. So, in November 1951, Doll and Hill sent questionnaires to all the doctors on the United Kingdom Medical Register, in the belief that this group might be cooperative and remain traceable in the foreseeable future. In fact, Doll would study this particular group for the next fifty years. A few months later, the American Cancer Society was recruiting 100,000 volunteers from all sections of the population for a similar study. Large numbers of healthy participants would have to die before there would be useful results, so both teams imagined that it would take years.

Meanwhile, Ernst Wynder, the doctor who had pre-empted Hill and Doll's publication in 1950, was now attempting to demonstrate directly that cigarette smoke could be a cause of cancer, at least in laboratory mice. In his laboratory, fifty carton batches of Lucky Strike were smoked rhythmically by machines which mimicked the human action, precipitating a tarry liquid into an array of glass beakers. This was then diluted and brushed three times a week across the shaved backs of eighty-six mice. More than half of those surviving the first year developed cancerous lesions on their backs. As Wynder wrote in *Cancer Research* in 1953, the 'suspected human carcinogen has thus been proven to be a carcinogen for a laboratory animal'. It was another piece of the case that was being built against smoking.

Having sent out their questionnaire, Doll and Hill followed the 40,000 doctors that responded, recording each death and searching for the cause. Two and a half years after beginning the study, by March 1954 there had been thirty-six lung cancer deaths among those male doctors over the age of 35. Even with such small numbers, the results were startling because each of these had previously been a smoker, whereas no non-smokers had died of the disease at all. Just as in their previous report, Doll and Hill had shown that the risk of developing lung cancer was about twenty times higher for those who smoked than those who did not. In June 1954, the American Cancer Society announced the results of a study that had been following 187,766 men aged between 50 and 69 for the previous two years. The results included the statistic that smokers on a pack or more a day had a death rate that was 75 per cent higher than non-smokers.

When the British Minister for Health, Iain McLeod, convened a press conference to announce the link between smoking and health, later in 1954, he smoked all the way through it.

৯৯

'Why me' is a common reaction to cancer, and is often mentioned in other memoirs. Yet Dad never asked it. Four and a half months after his diagnosis, I asked him why not, why it was that he felt no need to address this apparently fundamental question.

He said he thought that he had just been unlucky, that the cards had fallen against him, that he would no more be able to explain his fate than explain how a tossed coin lands.

He did acknowledge that he might have been subjected to risks. As a young man he had smoked, but he had given up when the tax on cigarettes increased in the late 1940s. He had also had some contact with industrial chemicals: he had been born, in 1928, to an engineer at Imperial Chemical Industries and a mother who had a Ph.D. in chemistry, and had lived, during his childhood, in a town where the smoke from the chemical plants blotted the sky. He had worked briefly in the labs in his university holidays. But he had lived on the other side of town from the plants and had taken precautions as a student.

Although these experiences might have increased his risk, he believed that he had succumbed to the disease because of pure bad luck. Why a molecule of smoke, or of an environmental chemical, or whatever else, had damaged a particular cell at some point in the past was down to unadulterated fate. The translation of risks into a tangible disease had much to do with, as he quoted, the 'slings and arrows of outrageous fortune'.

In 1954, in order to counter the mounting evidence and the declining sales of cigarettes, the major American manufacturers created the Tobacco Industry Research Committee, shrewdly recruiting the former president of the American Cancer Society, a scientist called Clarence Little, as its head. His oft-repeated line was that there was 'no convincing clinical or experimental evidence' to indict smoking as the cause of lung cancer, and that 'unreasoning fear based on incomplete information is not a constructive force'. Although grants were made to independent investigators, they soon found that these were withdrawn when they discovered results that ran contrary to this prevailing idea.

Wilhelm Hueper added to this controversy by denying that cigarettes could be causing the lung cancer epidemic. 'The acceptance of the cigarette theory would require the extermination of a great deal of factual medical knowledge,' he wrote, bemoaning how smoke was obscuring his own work on industrial chemicals. Even as more and more evidence against cigarettes was amassed during the second half of the 1950s, he wrote scathing reviews of the available literature, accusing Doll and his colleagues of making 'extravagant claims' and 'contentions' that contained 'serious errors'. Doubting Doll's statistics, he suggested that other factors, such as smokers living in poor neighbourhoods or working in poisonous factories, had not been ruled out as a cause of the epidemic. In other scientific papers, he barely mentioned the possibility that cigarettes might be dangerous. 'He was German, he had absolutely no concept of statistical analysis,' remembered Doll. 'He had the German attitude to science which is one case proves a rule.'

There was something of a caged animal about Hueper during the 1950s; prevented from meeting patients, he spent his workdays dabbing cancer-causing chemicals such as uranium, nickel and chromate on to animals. Every year he announced another public danger, including pesticides, city smog and nickel, at a press conference or in front of a congressional committee. Although the Tobacco Industry Research Committee offered Hueper hundreds of thousands of dollars, he said that his science was not for sale.

In 1955, Ed Morrow anchored an American current affairs programme about the tobacco controversy, which canvassed opinion evenly from both sides of the debate, including from Wilhelm Hueper; Morrow himself smoked throughout.

In 1956, Doll and Hill reported the results from following their cohort of 40,000 doctors for fifty-three months: eighty-one had so far died of lung cancer, and once again the risk to heavy smokers was twenty times higher than those who had never touched a cigarette. The following year, the American Cancer Society survey of nearly 200,000 individuals produced yet more of the same: those who smoked two packs a day had sixty-four times the likelihood of dying than non-smokers; those smokers who gave up dramatically reduced their chances of dying within a few years of quitting; perhaps most tellingly, of the 448 lung cancer victims only fifteen had never smoked. In just seven years, the body of evidence against cigarettes had become almost overwhelming.

Yet just as the argument appeared to be flowing irrevocably against Hueper and his idea of environmental cancer, he found an eloquent ally.

In January 1958, Rachel Carson received a letter in which a friend called Olga Owens Huckins complained that the private bird sanctuary that she managed with her husband had been decimated by the pesticides sprayed from aeroplanes on to the surrounding fields. 'I then realized,' wrote Carson in *Silent Spring*, 'that I must write this book.' Fifty-one-year-old Carson was a biologist by training who had been a full-time writer about the natural world for the previous six years since her book *The Sea Around Us* had sold 200,000 copies. Although she was not naturally a campaigner, she felt compelled to defend nature from malign human interference. During the following two years, she travelled from Texas to Nova Scotia and spent some time with Wilhelm Hueper in Bethesda, to research the book. Hueper found her to be 'a sincere, unusually well-informed scientist possessing not only an unusual degree of social responsibility but also having the courage and ability to express and fight for her convictions and principles'.

Just as she was completing the cancer chapter of *Silent Spring*, in March 1960, she discovered lumps in her breasts. A few weeks later, at the Doctors Hospital in Washington, surgeons discovered a tumour in her left breast that was 'apparently benign' while in the other was a tumour 'suspicious enough to require a radical mastectomy', which was duly performed. She was not told of the full extent of her malignancy, as was normal practice at that time, something justified by doctors with the argument that patients might descend into despondency on hearing their full diagnosis. And, as a typical cancer patient of her time, she accepted her doctor's advice, told virtually nobody about her illness and certainly did not write about her ordeal. A cancer diagnosis was particularly hard because it promised an imminent death. Moreover, in the post-war years it signalled a malingering, repressed and melancholic personality, as many people still believed that the cause was psychological.

In November that year, some seven months after her diagnosis, Carson discovered that a 'curious, hard swelling [had] appeared on the 3rd and 4th rib on the operated side, at or near the junction to the sternum', which X-rays revealed to be located between the skin and the ribs. A few weeks later, she began a course of radiation therapy but continued to decline.

Silent Spring was published in the *New Yorker*, in the spring of 1962, two years after her cancer diagnosis. A few months later, the book was published, selling hundreds of thousands of copies in the US and elsewhere. The chapter on cancer ends with the stirring endorsement: 'Among the most eminent men in cancer research are many who share Dr Hueper's belief that malignant diseases can be reduced significantly by determined efforts to identify environmental causes and to eliminate them or reduce their impact.'

Although Carson's legacy was to be the birth of the environmental movement, her contribution to the debate about the causes of the rising cancer epidemic was, however, decidedly partisan. The flaw in her argument was that, in fact, this was not an epidemic of all cancers, but almost entirely consisted of those occurring in the lung, the number of deaths from which had risen in America from 3,000 in

1930 to 41,000 in 1962; numbers of deaths from other sorts of cancers had not similarly exploded. Yet in her chapter about cancer, Rachel Carson makes no mention of the risks of smoking or the growing body of evidence created by Richard Doll and his colleagues.

In 1962, in the midst of this ferocious debate, the US Surgeon General established a Committee on Smoking. The independent panel of eight doctors, comprising professors from established medical schools, a statistician and an organic chemist, had weighed the evidence, including the study of 40,000 British doctors and the scientific papers by Ernst Wynder, and had interrogated more than a hundred eminent researchers, Richard Doll and Wilhelm Hueper among them. The committee reported its unequivocal conclusion, in January 1964, that 'Cigarette smoking is associated with 70 per cent increase in the age specific death rates of males', and that it caused cancer. The press conference was held on a Saturday, so that the results would not unduly damage the stock market. Although some other countries, such as Britain, had reached such a consensual position a few years before, the Surgeon General's report marked a watershed everywhere. The universal belief in the danger of cigarettes can be traced back to that moment.

Amid the report's 386 pages, there was a detailed discussion of whether or not industrial carcinogens, pesticides or urban pollution could explain the increase in lung cancer. In turn, each one was dismissed. In particular, Hueper's theory about the dangers of industrial chemicals was rejected: 'It must be emphasized quite strongly that the population exposed to industrial carcinogens is relatively small and that these agents cannot account for the increasing lung cancer risk in the general population.'

In April 1964, four years after her diagnosis, Rachel Carson had one final surgical procedure. When this failed to stem the disease, she was returned home and died a few days later.

Wilhelm Hueper retired later that year. The section of the National Cancer Institute that he had headed was disbanded; his carefully collected library was dispersed. 'I left the National Cancer Institute with the impression that I had not succeeded in laying a foundation through my work, on which others might erect a solid building,' he wrote.

❧

In the summer of 2004, I travelled to Oxford to meet Richard Doll. As my father so admired him, this particular interview felt as if it had some special importance. I had tried to meet Doll a month earlier, but he told me that he would be much too busy. I had not been entirely certain what could detain a 92-year-old, until I read the reports of his fifty-year follow-up of his study of 40,000 British doctors, which were published in every newspaper during that month. Unsurprisingly, it contained yet more evidence for the perniciousness of smoke.

Doll had white hair and a slight stoop, but his passion had been undimmed by age. He was also a much funnier interviewee than most, mixing his campaigning zeal with wry and cheeky jokes directed mostly against his more pompous colleagues. Before I had a chance to sit down and set up my tape recorder, he pulled out *The Causes of Cancer*, a book that he had written with a colleague called Richard Peto some years before. With great urgency and intensity, Doll explained how this report demonstrated that pesticides, food colourings, herbicides and fertilisers found in small traces in the environment were not responsible for the rise in cancer death rates during the twentieth century. The battle that had begun with Hueper and others in the middle of the twentieth century clearly remained very much alive. Even during tea, an hour and a half later, Doll returned to the subject, clearly believing that one of his priorities was to destroy what he saw as the myth of environmental cancer. I don't think he understood why I was writing a book about the past when there was so much to fight for in the future. He died in July 2005.

&

Although the causes of cancer remain a disputed topic, the medical establishment – which includes the major cancer research organisations in Britain and America and many doctors – speaks with one voice. For them, the largest single reason for the rise of cancer deaths during the twentieth century is smoking. Today, of the 10 million cancers diagnosed each year throughout the world about a third of them are the result of chewing and smoking tobacco, with tumours arising not only in the lungs but also in the mouth and airways, and in the pancreas, kidney and bladder as the toxins are transported in the blood. Although this number is enormous, it would have been much larger without the work of Richard Doll and his colleagues in the 1950s, which inspired a campaign to control tobacco and encouraged the population to give up or not to begin at all. Indeed, now only between 20 and 30 per cent of the population in Europe and America continue to smoke compared to the 66 per cent who smoked shortly after the Second World War; although young women in particular seem reluctant to adopt the health promotion messages. The campaign to control tobacco was, therefore, one of the most significant contributions to public health, at least in western countries, the twentieth century.

Pesticides are, by contrast, a much weaker threat to the population as a whole, although agricultural workers who suffer high and repeated doses can develop cancer. Most scientists now doubt the truth of Rachel Carson's statement 'Man has put the vast majority of carcinogens into the environment, and he can, if he wishes, eliminate many of them.' One flaw in her argument, many scientists believe, is that the human body has always had to deal with traces of environmental chemicals, from the smoke in primeval huts and the tar that our ancestors painted their boats with, to the charred meat that they ate.

Moreover, the natural world is full of chemicals that cause cancer, which are very similar to their man-made counterparts. Fruit and vegetables such as bananas, basil, broccoli, lettuce, parsley and turnips contain natural pesticides in order to ward off predators, which when dabbed on the backs of mice also create cancer. A typical human diet contains natural carcinogens at one thousand times the quantities of the traces of artificial contaminants. So although there may be small, marginal risks from low levels of industrial chemicals in the environment, they pale into insignificance compared to other risks. As a consequence of this and other studies, neither the American Cancer Society nor Cancer Research UK warn against the cancer dangers of pesticides in the food chain. By contrast, industrial and agricultural chemicals, when used repeatedly by those who work with them, do contribute to between about 5 and 10 per cent of all cancers, according to Doll's study. And these could be prevented relatively simply.

In *The Causes of Cancer*, Doll and his colleague Richard Peto assert that the second major cause of cancer is diet, which is charged with about a third of all cancers. Many other studies have shown that increased consumption of red meat, in particular, appears to be associated with rising levels of colon cancer, although scientists are not quite sure why. One theory is that cooking red meat at high temperatures produces various carcinogens; one experiment showed that a burger that was flipped once a minute created less of a carcinogen called 'heterocyclic amine' than a burger that was turned only once during cooking, allowing it to become dark and charred. Similarly, fat dripping from barbecuing steaks is fired back up from the charcoal as a carcinogenic smoke, which coats the meat.

In addition, a diet lacking in certain sorts of vegetables may also be a contributing factor: plant chemicals, often found in cruciferous vegetables such as broccoli, kohlrabi and fennel, contribute to the health of cells. These chemicals bind to potentially dangerous carcinogens within cells, thereby preventing genetic damage. And other vegetable constituents may help cells to repair strings of DNA that have become damaged in some way.

Yet the triggers of cancer arise not only from the intake of chemicals of various types, including those found in cigarettes; they are as diverse as the forms of the disease: a bacteria called Helicobacter pylori, which resides in the ferocious acid of the stomach, can spark it; and the naturally occurring female hormone called oestrogen seems to encourage some breast tumours to grow.

The love affair with the sun tan, promoted by icons such as Coco Chanel and Rita Hayworth in the 1930s and 1940s, also created one of the fastest growing cancer epidemics of the century. In some countries incident rates of malignant melanoma, the most malicious skin cancer, were increasing by as much as 5 per cent a year by the 1970s, although this rate of growth has abated somewhat with growing public awareness. Nonetheless, beaches everywhere remain packed with sunbathers repeatedly damaging their skin cells.

In addition, the creation of human society probably contributed to the onset of the disease as our behaviour as a species is so different to that of early man. Our cells were created over several million years to meet the challenges of hunting and gathering and of living to a certain age. Now, we live much longer, with less exercise and greater access to food. 'It may seem extraordinary that something as simple as too many calories and too much oxygen-fuelled activity in our cells could be a major factor in cancer risk – but it makes sense,' writes Professor Mel Greaves, in *Cancer: The Evolutionary Legacy*. When rats have their calorie intake reduced, for example, their cancer rates decline.

Similarly, some of the causes of breast cancer probably have their roots deep in a past in which women evolved to have a monthly menstrual cycle. This was very different from the reproductive cycles of other animals, which only have short periods of fertility in certain seasons. As a consequence, childbearing began early and continued without much interruption until menopause. Moreover, today's women face many more menstrual cycles as their lives are less interrupted by pregnancy. As a result, the female body is bathed in more hormones, including oestrogen, which encourage cells in the breast to proliferate in expectation of pregnancy. Not only does this encourage nascent tumours to develop, but each time a cell divides there is a danger that it will mutate into a malignancy. It is now understood that the nuns of Bernardino Ramazzini's 1700 study, who were more susceptible to breast cancer than other women, were fighting these evolutionary forces.

Today, one in three people will develop cancer in their lifetime, a larger proportion even than when Rachel Carson wrote her book. The reason for this increase is unlikely to be the industrial and agricultural chemicals, lying like a patina across our lives, which she deemed the major threat. Rather it is the result of our changing lives and behaviour. Paradoxically, because we suffer less from other diseases and we live richer lives, we are more likely to develop cancer.

❦

Five months after his diagnosis, Dad embraced life with still greater ferocity. As if only the present existed, and refusing to look beyond, he rushed to plays, concerts and exhibitions. Even before he was properly healthy, he was being pushed around in a wheelchair by Mum at a Picasso exhibition. With the return of his vitality, there was little to stop him. In those months of health, as the memories of his bloody operation receded, I happily thought the old Dad was returning, unaware that he felt a new-found urgency. I saw him when he travelled the two hours to London for concerts, lectures or a trip to an art gallery. In the early evenings of those trips, I met him for a swift dinner, and then he would rush off into the night towards another performance, thrusting his hand into the air with his characteristic wave, without a backward glance. Witty and sarcastic, he would chastise my friends for their insufficient grasp of history, and joke about our lives. They all drank to his health.

Chemotherapy:
the hunt for the magic bullet

WITH DAD SO APPARENTLY HEALTHY, I thought there was no need to travel the two hours to Birmingham for his seventy-fourth birthday party. It was seven months after the diagnosis. I made myself believe there would be so many other birthdays for me to attend. But a few weeks later, I went to visit him. At dinner, Jessica, my niece, Dad's first grand-daughter, aged almost 4, put her finger to her lips, 'shhh', as if we had to follow her nursery-school's dinner-table rules. 'Nobody is allowed to say anything,' she said. After the interruption, Dad talked about an article he'd seen in the newspaper. 'Beeee quiiiiettt,' she shouted. As he continued, enormous droplets welled up in her eyes, her lips turned downwards, then tears rolled down her cheeks.

❧

I find it difficult not to superimpose the image of Jessica upon the 4-year-old girl who was admitted to Boston Children's Hospital, in February 1947. Her name was not given in the case report. Tired and pale, she suffered from aching bones and bruised easily. Pressing her belly, a doctor found that her spleen was enormously swollen, and drew blood for tests. Another pushed a needle into her sternum's bone marrow – a procedure creating enormous pain. According to one of her doctors, the needles themselves were of such poor quality that he sharpened them himself and kept a pair of pliers on hand in case they broke off and needed to be pulled out of a child's chest.

In the pathology laboratory, a few floors away, her blood was examined and found to be littered with large, misshapen white blood cells. The diagnosis was acute leukaemia, and the prognosis was a painful life of between three and five months, little having changed since Rudolf Virchow first identified the disease a century before, in Berlin. So harrowing was the work of telling parents these facts, that childhood oncology was a particularly unpopular speciality among doctors. The standard procedure was to send these children home to die in peace.

Sidney Farber was the head of pathology at Boston Children's Hospital at the time. Aged 43, he had spent the previous seventeen years studying the blood, bone and flesh of patients who were in the care of the hospital, producing a series of robust, if not terribly innovative, scientific reports. Always formal, addressing his colleagues only by their surnames, he preferred the laboratory to the frontline of the wards. When he did meet patients he perfectly enacted the Galenic role of a physician – patrician, supremely confident, with an easy authority and always dressed in perfectly tailored suits.

Although many scientists were despondent, believing that research into a cure for leukaemia was futile, Sidney Farber cherished a hope that a chemical would be found to kill cancer cells. While a few others shared these ideas, they were on the fringes of the medical community. 'In the minds of most physicians,' one wrote, 'the administration of drugs other than analgesic [painkilling] in the treatment of malignant disease was the act of a charlatan.' There had been one report from Yale in which a chemical had appeared to prolong the lives of a few sufferers with lymphoma, but overall most doctors thought that it was unlikely that some agent would kill only cancerous cells while leaving the healthy body intact; patients invited to try out these new potential drugs, therefore, would surely suffer horribly, without seeing any improvement in their disease.

Some days after arriving in hospital, the 4-year-old girl appeared to be reaching the final act of her illness. But Farber had just received a vial of a yellow-orange powder from the Lederle Laboratories in Pearl River, New York. The powder was one member of a family of chemicals called 'folic acid antagonists', which blocked folic acid, a recently discovered chemical that was thought not only to be responsible for the colour of butterfly wings, but also to play an essential part in the mechanism by which cells divide. Farber hoped that the powder would slow down the speed at which the girl's cells replicated, thereby retarding her cancer – although his choice of agent had as much to do with intuition as rigorous analysis.

On 28 March, Farber ordered that 40 mg of the substance be injected into her thigh muscle. As it coursed through her body, it caused pain. In later cases, with this class of drug, most patients vomited, soon after injection, as if their bodies were desperately trying to clear their systems. The following day another dose was injected, but the drug did little to mitigate the disease. Her inexorable decline continued, the pain increasing. The skin of her gums and intestines became cracked and haemorrhaged blood. Yet every day, for a week, the drug was injected.

The atmosphere of the Children's Hospital in the late 1940s was somewhat forbidding, the doctors a little formal and aloof. Only parents were allowed to visit the child patients, siblings and other relations often reduced to waving from the courtyard.

A week after the girl's treatment had begun, she died of what was presumed to be the normal course of the leukaemia. Her tiny body was carried to the mortuary, then her blood and bone samples were taken to Farber's pathology laboratory. Remarkably, the bone marrow contained only a few immature leukaemic cells. 'A change of this magnitude in such a short time,' wrote Farber, 'has not been encountered ... in our experience.' It was a germ of hope for other children.

The breakthrough with the girl now inspired Farber to continue the experiment. Five days after her death, a 7-year-old boy – referred to by the initials W.G. in the case report – entered the hospital. A few months before, he had noticed a pain in his knee, which had travelled to his elbow and now migrated randomly around his body. Although the doctor examining him noted a slight enlargement of his spleen and liver, the boy appeared to be 'well developed and nourished and not particularly ill'. The laboratory report, however, was unequivocal: he had 56,000 white blood cells per cubic millimetre of blood, about a drop, which was about ten times more than normal; of these, 73 per cent were diseased. The bone marrow biopsy told the same story.

One week after admittance, Farber began to treat W.G. with the same folic acid antagonist that seemed to have achieved something for the girl. Although W.G. felt the pain and nausea from the chemical, he remained active and was soon discharged, first to a convalescent home and then to his own. But behind this apparently healthy façade, W.G.'s body was disintegrating: his white blood cell count remained high, and his red blood cells were becoming scarcer.

With that treatment failing, Farber reached for another of the half dozen or so folic acid antagonists which the Lederle Laboratories had produced. He had instructed them to produce a range, in the hope that one would block folic acid's action in leukaemic cells; it was like searching through a collection of differently shaped keys in the hope that one might fit a pre-existing lock.

The second folic acid antagonist had side effects no

less harrowing. In any case, day by day, W.G. declined; his stomach grew firm as his liver and spleen swelled abnormally and, with fewer and fewer red blood cells circulating through his body, he became breathless and pallid. A few times a week, he travelled from home to the hospital, where Farber's doctors painfully took his blood and bone marrow samples. Four months after admission, 94 per cent of his white blood cells were diseased. A few days later, on 13 August 1947, as his temperature rose to the nearly fatal 106 °F, he was rushed back to hospital where he was resuscitated with several blood transfusions.

During the four months that Farber had been treating W.G., he had also recruited a handful of other patients to his experiment, although it had not always been easy to persuade their parents to consent. All these experimental subjects were suffering and some had died by the time W.G. returned to hospital. Nonetheless, Farber single-mindedly called for more children and more chemicals. The junior doctors on the ward, however, were becoming increasingly angered by the children's day-to-day suffering, which they were experiencing at first-hand. Complaining to the head of paediatrics, Charles Janeway, they demanded that the children be allowed to die peacefully, away from the long needles and toxic chemicals. They objected to Farber's seemingly cruel experiments and his aloof manner, there being little more than a hopeful hypothesis to suggest that the drugs would ever lead to anything beneficial. For some time, these junior doctors conducted warfare against the five members of Farber's experimental team, obstructing their work with the children. Demanding and, at times, a difficult man to work with, Farber did not respond to this crisis with good grace; but eventually Janeway talked with Farber and his colleagues and, having satisfied himself that the research was worthwhile, convinced his subordinates to cooperate.

It was now five months after W.G.'s initial diagnosis and after the blood transfusions his life was no longer endangered. So Farber began him on another combination of folic acid antagonists and within two weeks he had recovered sufficiently to be discharged. But every day he returned to what was grandly named the hospital's Tumour Therapy Office – an inhospitable vestibule connected to the men's toilet, with a corridor for a waiting room – where his blood was tested, and the drugs were injected. By now, the nausea and the pain were, at least, expected. He began slowly to climb back towards health: his liver and spleen diminished in size, and he began to eat more heartily. Six weeks after his near-fatal collapse, he returned to be among his classmates at school. Nobody knew, however, whether this was the effect of the drugs or if this was the ebb and flow of the disease, as leukaemia patients occasionally recovered somewhat only to relapse again.

The relief his family felt lasted barely a month; thereafter, he deteriorated quite rapidly, his liver and spleen growing every day. Despite Sidney Farber's good intentions, this latest folic acid antagonist, the fourth attempt, was failing. At crisis point once again, blood transfusions saved W.G. from death. It was seven and a half months after first admission. Determined, Farber offered W.G. yet another drug, this one called aminopterin. There remained only a last faint hope.

W.G. received daily injections in the thigh beginning on Tuesday 16 December 1947. Every day, for six days, he returned for a dose and blood tests. And slowly but perceptibly, his white blood count – which had been 60,000 white cells per droplet – began to decline, his appetite returning in time for his family's Christmas festivities. When he returned to hospital on 30 December, fourteen days after the course of therapy had begun, there were 19,000 white blood cells per droplet – about double the healthy range but an enormous improvement. For the first time a folic acid antagonist seemed to be having a direct effect. But W.G. was prevented from his daily hospital visits because some of the worst snowfalls in recent history now blocked the roads.

Just before the New Year, a 2-year-old boy was brought to the Tumour Therapy Office. An identical twin, he was already unable to walk whilst his brother remained in good health. The previous month, the patient had been admitted to hospital with arthritis and an infection of his windpipe; his body was pocked with bruises and his gums oozed pus. His white blood cell count stood at 60,000 per cubic millimetre, on 28 December. Farber prescribed a dose of aminopterin. The following day, his blood count had already fallen. After three daily doses, it had reached 9,000 – the upper end of the normal range. Yet despite the improvement, his respiratory infection worsened on New Year's Eve, making it difficult for him to breathe. His doctors stopped the aminopterin and admitted him to hospital where he was given a transfusion. Four days later, he had recovered and was discharged with a white blood count now down to 2,700. When he returned to the Tumour Therapy Office, ten days later, he was transformed: his appetite was ravenous, he was walking for the first time in two months, he could breathe freely, there was no more bleeding and his spleen had shrunk, decreasing the size of his stomach to such an extent that his clothes now hung loosely.

Nobody had ever seen such a response. Then a two-and-a-half-year-old girl with leukaemia was put on the drug, and within two weeks she began to 'play and run like a normal child'. With her parents reporting that she was now more active than ever, the doctors on the children's oncology ward finally began to participate enthusiastically in Farber's research.

After the snows melted, W.G. returned to hospital on 3 February 1948. Although he had received small doses of the drug from his family doctor while at home, his white blood cell count had risen. Within ten days of returning to the Tumour Therapy Office, however, he was showing a marked improvement, his white blood cell count falling from 78,000 to 5,000. But as the daily dose continued, his gums began to ooze with pus and blood. Dr Robert Mercer, the member of Farber's team who spent the most time with patients, suggested to Farber that these were the toxic side effects of the drug itself. But Farber refused to listen: he believed that his wonder drug was benign, and that the damage was being caused naturally by the leukaemia itself. Yet as the symptoms persisted, inflicting more pain on W.G., Mercer grew more reluctant to administer the drug. To resolve the matter, he demanded that Farber examine W.G. so that he could see the damage for himself. Farber rebuked Mercer who, he suggested, was suffering from the remnants of some kind of Second World War battle fatigue. Yet within a day or two, Farber conceded, suspending W.G.'s daily doses for a week in order to allow his gums to heal. Within a few weeks, he was, as Farber put it, 'in excellent physical condition'.

Sidney Farber presented a report of his research at a meeting of local doctors at the Boston Children's Medical Center, on 8 April 1948. Describing in detail six of the cases who had their lives extended because of the drug, he also said that of the sixteen children he had treated since W.G.'s first dose four months previously, ten had improved. Of the six that had not responded, four were already dead. Farber himself remained optimistic yet cautious, as it was uncertain how long these remissions might last. For many of the audience, the results went against their intuition. Scepticism and incredulity reigned, remembered Farber's colleague Robert Mercer, who was also there, some of the doctors even refusing to discuss the paper with Farber fearing that he had 'gone round the bend'.

For others, though, the news from Boston offered some hope. Soon Farber began to receive letters, telephone calls and telegrams referring patients to him or asking for some aminopterin. When the report was published, in the *New England Journal of Medicine*, a few months later, the demand for information became so intense that Farber had to organise a series of large seminars to inform as many doctors as possible of his findings. Although Farber had been careful not to promise a cure, the newspaper reports implied that he had. A week after he had delivered the paper in Boston, for example, the Associated Press issued a wire story with the headline 'NAVY FLYING SICK CHILD' about a patient from San Diego being airlifted to Sidney Farber: 'The child is Linda Dias, three years old, dying with Leukemia. She will be treated at the Boston Children's Hospital with a recently discovered drug aminopterin. Doctors here had recently given up hope for her.'

The intense public reaction to Farber's results was, in part, because cancer was once again meriting attention, after a period during the war where other concerns were deemed to be more important. With the cancer death rate continuing to rise, President Truman had declared that April, the very month of Farber's announcement, was to be 'cancer control month'. At much the same time, two industrialists, Alfred Sloan and Charles Kettering, respectively the chairman and head of research of General Motors, had donated $4 million in order to build, in New York, the largest privately funded cancer research institute in the world. 'Very rapid progress against this mysterious scourge could be made possible,' said Sloan as he opened the fourteen-storey building, 'if the problem got the same amount of money, brains and planning that was devoted to the atomic bomb.' The *New York Times* reported the event with the headline, 'C-DAY LANDING WON IN WAR ON CANCER'.

Public interest reached even greater heights that August with the death from a neck tumour of Babe Ruth, the former New York Yankees baseball star. In the days preceding it, the public had swamped Memorial Hospital staff with 13,000 letters and telegrams of support. His obituaries praised his courage in fighting the 'scourge that kills more than 170,000 Americans every year and is responsible for one out of eight deaths'. Days later, it was also revealed that his doctor had innovatively tested a chemical treatment – albeit not a folic acid antagonist – on the Sultan of Swat, as he was known, during the previous year, making Farber's endeavour all the more significant.

❦

Six months after Dad's operation to rebuild his neck and excise the cancer, my parents and a few of their friends planned a short winter break in Paris, as a celebration of his new-found health and a nostalgic remembrance of the early days of their marriage. A week before they left, however, he felt a terrible pain in his stomach and was rushed into hospital. Fearing another tumour, we were relieved when it turned out to be just some kind of painful but solvable intestinal obstruction. The scare simply hardened his determination to travel.

The night before departure, Dad came to dinner; he was cheery, there was a new sparkle in his eyes and a cheekiness in his conversation. In Paris, he discovered new reserves of energy which inspired him to walk all over the city, eat at a newly renovated Art Deco brasserie, go to the theatre and see a Constable exhibition that had been curated by Lucian Freud. He even visited an archaic type-foundry, was given a tour of their ancient machines, which poured molten lead into letter-shaped moulds, and ordered a font of ornamental type that he hoped he would be able to use in his next printing project. He also learnt the idiom '*C'est pas la mer à boire*' (it is not the sea to drink) which means something like 'it's no big deal'.

On his final day, he remained in one last gallery a little too long so that, in danger of missing the train back to England, he had to run across town. On the way home, he noticed that one of his hips ached. He presumed it was just that he had become so unaccustomed to so much activity. '*C'est pas la mer à boire*,' he said.

By the early 1950s, Farber believed that he had proved in principle that cancer 'chemotherapy' worked. For the first time, patients were living with – albeit not for very long – rather than dying quickly of leukaemia. In one scientific paper, Farber announced that W.G. was still alive twenty-three months after the onset of disease; the 2-year-old boy also remained as strong and healthy as his twin sixteen months after diagnosis. In the end, though, most chemotherapy patients relapsed as the tumour developed resistance to the drug.

The successes of the first patients, Farber believed, also had therapeutic benefits for others: 'If the entire atmosphere is guarded optimism based upon actual achievement in laboratory research,' Farber wrote, 'then fear is more easily dispelled and replaced by courageous handling of problems.' The economist J. K. Galbraith wrote that Farber 'never allowed us to give up hope' when his youngest son was treated for leukaemia at this time.

In addition, as the discoverer of the first new weapon in the anti-cancer armoury in two generations, Farber was thrown into the heart of American life, using his celebrity to raise money by appearing on nationwide radio shows or at dinners with the baseball team the Boston Red Sox.

Driven by these first successes, Farber's ambition hardened. He now believed that a cure for all cancers, from lung to breast, stomach to skin, was possible. All that was required to discover this new range of chemotherapies was sufficient resources and a systematic programme; and the only institution able to do so, with enough power and money, was Government. Whereas the National Institutes for Health had previously funded an eclectic mix of research programmes – some investigating the basic workings of the cell, others attempting to discover treatments – Farber demanded a concerted effort to speedily create new chemotherapy drugs.

'I think it is sad indeed that chemical compounds which might conceivably be of great help to patients now having cancer cannot be administered because there are not enough teams and facilities to do it,' said Farber in the early 1950s, believing that it should be possible for thousands more chemicals to be tested each year. Fast becoming a slick political operator, Farber found allies in this crusade.

Dr Cornelius Rhoads was the first director of research at the Sloan-Kettering Institute. During the war, Rhoads had been the head of the American Government's Chemical Warfare Division, which had itself accidentally provided some of the first evidence that chemotherapy might be successful. On 2 December 1943, a fleet of German planes had dropped bombs on seventeen Allied ships crowded into the Italian port of Bari. One ship, the *John Harvey*, which was loaded with tons of mustard gas, took a direct hit. So much gas billowed into the air that even the water turned acidic. Yet so secret was the cargo, the gas never having been used during the war, that none of the medical personnel treating the survivors had realised that many of their patients were suffering the effects of gas poisoning. As many huddled in their toxin-sodden clothes, they therefore absorbed the full force of the chemical rather than showering it off. By the end of that night, sixty-nine seamen had died from the effects of the gas and a further 600 had been severely affected. Autopsies revealed that the gas had atrophied their lymph nodes and spleens – a terrible if remarkable finding which demonstrated that chemicals can discriminate, selectively destroying parts of the body rather than the whole. And importantly, the organs affected were exactly those damaged by leukaemia.

Just when Farber was succeeding with aminopterin, Rhoads had employed many of the staff of the Chemical Warfare Division and moved some of its equipment to the Sloan-Kettering Institute's thirteenth floor. He was known for charging about the institute's corridors, periodically shouting 'chicks' – his shorthand for secretaries. He believed passionately that Government should fund a systematic search for chemotherapy drugs, which would be reminiscent of the wartime efforts that had brought together large numbers of scientists in order to hasten the testing and production of penicillin and anti-malarial drugs. Together with Farber, he lobbied the administrators of the National Institutes of Health and their political masters, both appearing at a series of Senate and congressional committees to press their case.

The third member of this campaigning triumvirate was Mary Lasker, a wealthy widow who lived in a six-storey townhouse on the Upper East Side of New York – a house packed with her collection of Matisses, Picassos and Monets – and who was then devoting much of her time and money to campaigning for public health initiatives and more medical research. Her interest in cancer, she said, stemmed from her seeing, as a young child, her mother's laundress after a double mastectomy. That Lasker's own husband Albert had succumbed to colon cancer in 1952 gave a strong personal edge to her determination. He had made his fortune as the advertising executive who had dreamed up the slogan 'Reach for a Lucky Instead', which had made Lucky Strike cigarettes the brand leader in the 1920s. United in their frustration about the slow pace of cancer research, Farber often joked that he and Mary Lasker communicated via 'mental telepathy'.

Lasker contributed to Rhoads and Farber's campaign by funding some of their initial research, although even the $100,000 she supplied did not take the systematic programme of testing chemicals very far. At the same time, as she was usefully connected, she badgered the President and legislators in person. She recalled John F. Kennedy as 'this very, very skinny and very young-looking Congressman. He looked incredibly young. His arms were too long for his coat.' Another tactic she employed to gain influence was to bestow powerful Senate figures with the 'public service award' of the Albert Lasker Foundation.

At the Senate Appropriations' sub-committee in 1953, Farber brought along a slide show. One image was of a boy who was under treatment smiling towards the lens. 'This little fellow … has been on borrowed time now for 45 months, since the onset of treatment,' Farber said, 'and he is still in excellent condition. He is leading the way, and those working in the field believe that if it can be achieved in one then it must be achieved in others.'

Their efforts paid off, for after Eisenhower's inauguration, he asked Farber, Rhoads and Lasker to sit on the National Advisory Cancer Council. Now with seats at the Washington high table, they persuaded Congress, in 1953, to give a $3 million grant distributed through the National Cancer Institute to establish the National Cancer Chemotherapy Service. Managed by a series of committees on which Lasker, Farber and Rhoads sat, the Service contracted various researchers and institutions across America to carry out the task of testing more than 100,000 different chemicals – under the informal slogan 'nothing too stupid to test' – in the blind hope that a few might prove useful anti-cancer agents. This library of potential drugs was built up in every conceivable way: synthesised in the laboratory; borrowed from secret army research projects; sifted out of fungi and yeast; extracted from plants such as periwinkle and even from such animals as sea urchins. Each drug was then tested on mice, to discover how toxic it was and whether it had any anti-tumour effects. 'Inevitably as I see it, we can look forward to something like a Penicillin for cancer,' Dr Rhoads told the *New York Times*, 'I hope within the next decade.'

The belief that chemotherapy might, one day, cure all cancers was bolstered, in 1956, when two researchers, Roy Hertz and Min Chiu Li, from the National Cancer Institute, cured a woman with choriocarcinoma, a highly malignant cancer arising in the placenta of pregnant women, using a chemical called methotrexate. It was the first solid tumour to fall to the weapon of chemotherapy. To many, it demonstrated that many other solid tumours would also be cured by chemicals.

By 1957, chemotherapy drug testing had increased to such an extent that 100,000 mice were having to be bred each year. That year, Lasker, Rhoads and Farber also succeeded in increasing the budget for the National Cancer Chemotherapy Service to an annual $14.9 million. Two years later, it rose again to $31.4 million.

Five years after it began, the Chemotherapy Service could boast few successes, and many scientists were arguing for a re-allocation elsewhere of its enormous resources. One prominent critic called Alfred Gellhorn took these complaints to the National Advisory Cancer Council, on which Lasker and Farber sat. 'The mass and mechanized type of screening now employed,' he said, 'is less likely to be productive than the investigations of an individual investigator who is interested and alert.' Other researchers pointed out that many of the thirty or so drugs that the National Cancer Chemotherapy Service claimed to have discovered had, in fact, been found by drug companies and researchers outside their mechanisms. The failure proved, the critics claimed, that science was not susceptible to being managed like some engineering project; singular belief and discerning analysis were, with a modicum of luck, more likely to achieve results. Farber, however, believed that not enough chemicals were being tested fast enough to save patients' lives. In consequence, he persuaded the administration to boost the annual grant to $42 million, a third of the total federal spending on cancer research.

By 1960, the hope that chemotherapy would finally cure all cancers was already fast diminishing. That year Mary Lasker wrote of Cornelius Rhoads's recent death, stating, 'Still his burning ambition to find *the* cure for cancer had not been achieved. His crusade, in that sense, may have seemed a failure.'

In December, thirty-five weeks after Dad's diagnosis, I waited for my parents at a London station in order to drive them South to a Christmas lunch in Brighton. I saw Mum come through the ticket barriers laden with suitcases and bags. Labouring behind her, his weight supported by a walking stick, came Dad, his previously energetic strides replaced by a foot-dragging slog. Suddenly he was old. With some disappointment he remarked that he would now be treated by geriatricians, for no longer was he a patient of the bright young things of neurosurgery. Dad was tired throughout the Christmas party, drinking little. His voice no longer resonated around the room. And although his grandchildren, Danny and Jessica, ran around him, he could not muster the energy to pick them up. Mum whispered to me that during the previous week he had been in such pain he had been barely able to pull himself from the bed each morning.

As ever, Dad and I talked, but he had lost his contrarian's passion. His brain was sluggish. Those tiny facts that he used to be able to pull from the chaotic filing system of his mind were no longer available. I told him about Sidney Farber and Mary Lasker and the disappointment of the 1950s. When he said he understood what it must have felt like to dedicate oneself to an endeavour and to fail, I knew implicitly that he was talking about his struggle against the disease.

On visiting my flat the next day, he could barely summon the energy to climb the stairs. For fifteen long minutes, I watched as he dragged his way up, wheezing at every step.

When a chemotherapy drug – a chemical toxin – enters the body, as a tablet, capsule or through an injection, it disperses. Patients describe the sensation as being rather like fire seeping through their flesh. Molecules of the chemical reach cells throughout the body, from the toes to the tongue, as well as the site of the tumour, wherever that may be. When the drug reaches the stomach cells, it stimulates signals that instruct the brain to begin vomiting. Some modern chemotherapy drugs reduce this effect by interfering with these signals.

Not every molecule of a chemotherapy drug has an effect. Their force can be reduced by other chemicals which naturally exist in cells and circulate around the body. And in some cells, although the toxins cause damage these cells are able to repair themselves.

But in other cells the chemotherapy molecules fatally harm the structure of the cell or irreparably damage the details of the genetic mechanisms, after which the cell begins the process whereby it destroys itself – blemished, it commits suicide. Chemotherapy is powerful because its effect is dispro-portional on fast-duplicating cells, such as tumour cells. In addition, tumour cells are often unable to repair themselves because they have often sustained other kinds of damage.

There are other cells in the human body, such as those in the hair or in the lining of the stomach wall, which also duplicate at a faster rate than others, hence chemotherapy can result in hair loss or the development of ulcer-like symptoms.

While little was known about these mechanisms in the 1960s, doctors could see that their leukaemia patients had improved after chemotherapy. Yet unfortunately the disease would usually return after a few months or years. By studying mice, researchers realised that this was the result of the drugs killing large numbers of the cancerous cells but leaving some alive. As the less resilient cells had died, those that were left were stronger and more able to resist the chemical onslaught. After treatment, therefore, these stronger cells and their progeny were now better able to command more and more of the body's resources. And as they did so, the disease recurred. Much like the ebb and flow of species in a world dominated by the laws of Darwinian evolution chemotherapy kills off the less able cells but sets the stage for the resurgence of much more malicious species.

One answer was to use two different drugs. With each drug working slightly differently, the risk of resistant cells surviving and duplicating would be diminished, much as an animal would find it hard to cope simultaneously with less food *and* less warmth in its environment. Yet even with these so-called 'combination therapies', children relapsed – albeit after a few more months than with just a single drug.

In 1964, Howard Earle Skipper was working in the Southern Research Institute in Birmingham, Alabama. Although he had also been a member of the Chemical Warfare Division, he had chosen not to work with Cornelius Rhoads in New York. Rather, he had established a free-standing institute funded partly by the National Cancer Chemotherapy Service and partly by Alfred Sloan and Charles Kettering. Studying mice, he realised why childhood leukaemia had not been cured: doctors did not understand that they had to kill every last diseased cell in the body. The trouble was that patients were being given relatively low doses of chemo-therapy, and one dose did not kill a fixed number of cells but rather a proportion, leaving some cancerous cells alive. Imagine a garden overgrown with one species of bindweed; a single spray of herbicide will kill, say, 90 per cent of the plants. Every subsequent spray will kill a further 90 per cent of the remaining plants. But to leave just one bindweed plant alive risks the spread of its progeny throughout the garden. Skipper's research resulted in the creation of a treatment method, or protocol, of unprecedented force.

'We began wondering if we could *cure* Leukaemia rather than just treat it to gain temporary remission,' remembers Donald Pinkel, a protégé of Sidney Farber and the head of the children's cancer department at St Jude Hospital in Tennessee in the early 1960s. Aware of Skipper's research and the need to hunt down every single last cancerous cell,

Pinkel realised he would have to give high doses of chemotherapy drugs over longer periods of time, together with a combination of drugs so that a single cell would not become resistant. But even when he had adopted these methods, he found that his patients relapsed as a result of the leukaemia cells hidden in the brain and in the spinal fluid where blood-borne chemotherapies would never reach them. So Pinkel set out to target these recalcitrant cells by irradiating the brain and injecting chemotherapy into the spinal column: 'total therapy'.

James Eversull was only one and a half, in 1964, when he was diagnosed with leukaemia. His parents and grandmother travelled with him to the regional cancer centre at St Jude. His treatment began with the administration over six weeks of a cocktail of high doses of chemotherapy drugs. 'We had to convert what looked like a terminally ill patient into one who seemed to have at most an early stage of leukaemia,' said Pinkel. When James had recovered sufficiently, and was producing some healthy blood cells, he was given a week of daily doses of three further drugs. Afterwards, he received two weeks of radiation directly on to his brain and another chemotherapy drug injected into his spinal fluid. Other children were also put on the protocol. 'I remember the other children there,' he remembers. 'Screaming, whining and getting shots.' Such brute-force applications of treatments to such young bodies were unprecedented. Nausea, vomiting and an ulcerous mouth were the side effects. For the next year, James was kept on chemotherapy drugs. 'To stop chemotherapy could have meant death for the children,' remembered Pinkel.

But on 17 November 1966, James Eversull became the first child to be taken off the therapy. James never relapsed. Pinkel's strategy to kill each of the millions of leukaemia cells – in his blood, bone marrow, brain and spinal cord – had succeeded. Twenty-two years later, Eversull was still reported as leading a normal life.

In the years since these first cases, Pinkel and others adjusted the treatment protocols to the extent that about 80 per cent of children with leukaemia now survive for at least five years, many for years thereafter.

❧

Returning home after Christmas, I found Dad was much better. Suddenly he was busy, printing some cards for the Wynkyn de Worde Society, a lunch club for printers, publishers and book designers. Setting some type a couple of months before, he had described the experience as transcendent and now he was keen to finish the project. Not having the strength himself, he asked me to lift the heavy type frame into one of his Victorian presses. Then he stood for hours in front of the clattering machine, adjusting the ink levels and feeding in sheet after sheet of paper. Out of practice, he found himself frustratingly unable to reach the level of beauty and perfection that he had once achieved. His large hands once had the grace of an artisan, but now they seemed to be as clumsy as an amateur's. Standing at the threshold of the printing room, I watched him at work in his inky apron. It pleased me to see him return to his passion for the first time since his diagnosis.

The War on Cancer:
Richard Nixon's quest

O N 15 JULY 1969, Mary Lasker boarded American Airlines flight 463 from New York to Washington. As she often complained that the nation spent more on chewing gum than it did on cancer research, she was intent on fighting against the newly inaugurated President's talk of cutting health spending. Richard Nixon's proposals would reverse Lasker's hard-won gains of the previous twenty years, which had seen the budget of the National Cancer Institute rise from just about half a million to $181 million. While lesser operators might have been content merely to defend every dollar against cutbacks, Lasker was launching a pre-emptive strike: demanding both an unprecedented increase in funding and that Government should rigorously manage scientific research.

It was the day before Apollo 11's scheduled lift-off. As she made her way through the airports, the newspapers were packed with stories of how, just eight years before, President John F. Kennedy had committed the nation to landing a man on the moon. NASA was on the verge of achieving one of the most complex engineering feats of all time.

Lasker carried with her a document which demanded

that 'the same talents for organization, goal-directed, as have been used in outer space planning and financing should be applied to cancer'. She believed that if discipline, vigour and planning could be brought to many branches of the scientific endeavour, then cures would be quickly produced – just as NASA's successes were founded on the formulation of a coherent plan, with clear objectives and a predetermined critical path.

The proposal was for a radical departure from the way that science was currently practised, as Lasker had little patience with the meandering, chaotic process of discovery. She often complained that the scientific establishment favoured so-called basic research – such as investigating the mechanisms of cells, genes or viruses – rather than testing drugs or discovering vaccines in a clinical setting. In her impatience, she described the administrators of the National Institutes of Health as 'perverse', and afraid to 'bring medical science down to the patient'.

Lasker reached the office of Senator Ralph Yarborough, the then chairman of the Senate Committee of Labor and Public Welfare, a little before three that afternoon. During their discussion, she mentioned a book entitled *Cure for Cancer* by a Denver doctor called Solomon Garb which demanded that the search for a cure become a 'national goal' funded annually with $650 million – to be completed 'with the least possible delay'. Decades of arcane discoveries about the human cell, Garb argued and Lasker with him, could now be used as a launch pad for the final 'moon-shot' to a cure.

As the meeting drew to a close, Lasker came to the point: would Yarborough be willing to establish some kind of commission of independent experts, as a way of building a broad Washington consensus in favour of an enormous concerted programme to find a cancer cure? As a bolster to her pleas, Lasker had brought to the meeting a respected scientist from the Memorial Sloan-Kettering Hospital called Mathilde Krim, who was married to a political fund-raiser,

Arthur Krim, the former financial chair of the Democratic National Financial Committee. As further encouragement, each woman pledged $5,000 for Yarborough's upcoming senatorial election campaign, which was likely to be against a well-funded but little-known Texas congressman called George Bush. Lasker found Yarborough to be 'very, very disorganized and harassed', but he signed up to Lasker's plan.

Five days after Lasker's meeting with Yarborough, Neil Armstrong became the first man to walk on the moon. For Lasker, this showed that a concerted, well-funded and rigorously directed government project could achieve the seemingly impossible. And now she wanted similar methods applied to the quest for a cancer cure.

Passionate and still energetic at 69, Lasker campaigned as effectively in the corridors of power as she did in the salons of high society and the laboratories of medicine. 'It was such fun to see you in action. You are something!' the columnist Anne Landers told her about one such encounter. 'I have never seen such a combination of hard-sell and soft-sell – intertwined with charm – and levity – yet deadly serious.' Lasker was a friend of the former President Lyndon B. Johnson, and remained close to the Kennedy clan. And she ran a small foundation which organised annual awards for medical research, something she had instituted in honour of her late husband; scientists regarded these awards as nearly as prestigious as the Nobels. Her office also acted as a clearing house for information about cancer cures and kept her in touch with innovative scientists throughout the country.

Her annual Christmas party, held in her six-storey New York townhouse, included guests as diverse as Teddy Kennedy, Truman Capote, and the actors Lauren Bacall and Danny Kaye. As gossip columnists trilled about her dresses by Dior, Chanel and Givenchy (in hot-pink brocade or aqua chiffon), or how she had danced the night away to the music of a small orchestra, she would work the room, nurturing a network of contacts which her critics disparaged as 'Mary's Little Lambs'.

Two months after meeting Senator Yarborough, Mary Lasker returned from her holidays determined to begin building her Washington consensus in earnest. To take her message to Richard Nixon, she used well-placed friends. She lunched, for instance, at the Pentagon – the day before 250,000 people protested outside the building against Vietnam – with the secretary of defence, Melvin Laird, who as a congressman, had received the Lasker Award for public service six years previously. Then she and Sidney Farber met the pharmaceutical entrepreneur and long-time cancer campaigner Elmer Bobst, who was now part of Nixon's Kitchen Cabinet. Within a few months, both Bobst and Laird had informed her that they had raised her request for the establishment of a cancer commission with the President.

Lasker then paid $22,000 for a full-page advertisement in the *New York Times*; two-thirds of the page was taken up with the headline 'MR NIXON: YOU CAN CURE CANCER'. Below it, Farber had written, 'We are so close to a cure for cancer. We lack only the will and the kind of money and comprehensive planning that went into putting a man on the moon.' One corner of the page was printed with a coupon that could be cut out and sent to the President.

❧

Lasker's unquenchable belief that a cure could be discovered was founded on the growing success of chemotherapy in treating childhood leukaemia as pioneered by Sidney Farber. But she also placed much faith in a newly fashionable idea – albeit in a small but vocal part of the scientific community: that it might be possible to develop a vaccine which could prevent a range of cancers. Hopes were high, as, just a decade before, the polio vaccine had virtually eradicated the disease in the developed world. Now enthusiasts were predicting that a leukaemia vaccine could be readied within just a few years, presupposing, of course, that leukaemia was caused by a virus.

By the late 1960s, much was known about those viruses which caused polio, influenza or smallpox. Although viruses could not be seen by an optical microscope, with the commercialisation of the electron microscope, in 1965, lab workers were able to see them as tiny particles which breached cell walls. They had learnt that unlike larger human cells or even bacteria, which contain all the necessary ingredients for self-sustaining life, viruses are lifeless parasites that are only activated on entering host cells, where they strip off their outer coat and deliver a payload of deoxyribonucleic acid (DNA), which can then commandeer the cell's energy and resources to manufacture new viral particles. Eventually the host cell disintegrates, the virus particles bursting out, ready once again for new cells to penetrate. The destruction caused by the polio virus to the nerve cells of children leads to their paralysis. Scientists had also discovered that the active ingredients of viruses were genetic material – a few short fragments of DNA or its biological mirror, ribonucleic acid (RNA). 'A piece of bad news wrapped in protein' was how one Nobel Laureate described them.

By contrast, very little was known about human cancer viruses. The only solid evidence was the discovery in 1964 – in the laboratories of the Middlesex Hospital in London – of a virus that caused the very rare Burkitt's Lymphoma, a lymph cancer which only occurred in Africa. In addition, various other viruses had been discovered that caused tumours, leukaemia and lymphomas in chickens, mice and other animals. The mechanisms of these viruses, however, was hard to discern, as they lay beyond the resolution of even electron microscopes – although it was widely believed that when a cancer virus entered the cell it wrenched open the cell's DNA and inserted its own bad genes into the gap. Professors demonstrated this theory by first breaking the bakelite chains of the DNA models that sat on their desks, then inserting other sections of double helices into the void. The effect on cells was thought to be much like a robot going haywire after having been given the wrong instructions.

In order to discover the range of human cancer viruses and understand their mechanisms, the US Government's National Cancer Institute had embarked on the ambitious Special Virus Cancer Program (SVCP), which, by 1970, was costing $30 million a year in contracts for research. Lasker herself, when she had been a member of the institute's advisory board, had played a part in the project's formation, the centrepiece of which was Building 41, on the campus of the National Institutes of Health, in Bethesda, Maryland, which had cost $3.5 million. Designed to contain any potentially lethal pathogens that might be discovered, Building 41 was equipped with airlocks, anti-contamination chambers and rule-books requiring all employees to wear special-issue jumpsuits and to shower when passing from one zone to another. Widely displayed throughout Building 41 was the new biohazard sign of three interlocking circles on an orange background. The building was unveiled in 1969. The same year, Michael Crichton's *Andromeda Strain*, which depicted a similar facility, became a best-seller.

By the time Mary Lasker was promoting a concerted programme for a cancer cure, the Special Virus Cancer Program had instituted a mechanism of management much like Lasker had advocated for the totality of cancer medicine. Using flow charts, critical path analysis, a system of contracts, review groups and process engineers recruited from NASA, the project functioned as if its purpose was to build an aircraft carrier, rather than explore unknown regions of nature.

The virus cancer theory had been given a further boost in 1969 by a sprinkling of new discoveries: a survey of patients showed that some had already developed an immune response to a cancer virus, as if their bodies had already fought off an attack from a cancer-causing virus; and a virus particle was isolated from the brain of a young boy with cancer. In addition, two of the leaders of the Special Virus Cancer Program, George Todaro and Robert Huebner, developed a new hypothesis which speculated that most human cancers began when viruses which were dormant within the human body were brought alive by ageing, radiation and carcinogens. Though impossible to prove or demonstrate, this widely discussed new theory suggested that the Special Virus Cancer Program might hold the key to the cure of all cancers. Lasker promoted the idea to her network, sending people like Senator Yarborough press cuttings of stories such as the one that appeared in the *Saturday Evening Post* with Huebner on the front cover and the headline 'WILL THIS MAN CURE CANCER?'

෪

In the early spring of 1970, Lasker continued with her battle to establish a commission. Not content with badgering Yarborough, she sent telegrams to every single member of the relevant Senate committees, met with senators and congressmen, and distributed 10,000 bumper stickers bearing the slogan 'MR PRESIDENT. MEMBERS OF CONGRESS. PLEASE CURE CANCER'. The Senate soon passed a resolution, calling for the establishment of a 'National Panel of Consultants' who would recommend ways of conquering cancer by 1976 – in celebration of the American Bicentennial. Congress adopted a similar resolution, demanding a 'national crusade' with the same deadline, although there was hardly a scientist who believed it to be realistic. Lasker was somewhat to blame for this exuberance, for although she couched her most enthusiastic rhetoric with caveats, she also understood the power of a simple proposition. Politicians and policy makers were not interested, she argued, in arcane scientific discoveries or tentative messages. Rather, their adherence to populism required immediate medical advances of real benefit that could be straightforwardly communicated. Once a deadline had been set, neither she nor anyone else, therefore, did anything to disabuse politicians of the impossibility of its fulfilment.

As her campaign progressed, her hope was bolstered by new discoveries from the Special Virus Cancer Program, with various researchers reporting in June 1970 that they had identified virus particles in tumour samples. 'Scientists have found and photographed a virus that they believe is the cause of breast cancer,' reported the *Washington Post*. The next step was the vaccine.

In the early summer of 1970, Senator Yarborough asked Lasker to be the chair of the National Panel of Consultants, but she refused, thinking that someone else was more likely to attract 'serious attention'. Her choice was Benno Schmidt, who was a partner at the New York investment firm Whitney and Co., sat on the board of the Memorial Sloan-Kettering Hospital and had Republican affiliations, which, she hoped, might give the report more weight within the Nixon administration. Lasker also made suggestions to Yarborough for almost all the other members of the panel. Sidney Farber became the vice-chairman, and the rest of the twenty-four-strong committee mostly comprised her friends and long-time collaborators.

Throughout that autumn, she midwifed parts of a report called the 'National Program for the Conquest of Cancer', which was launched on 4 December 1970 in a committee room in the New Senate Office Building in Washington. The report read like a blueprint for a consistent and planned 'moon-shot' for cancer. Starting with the $180 million then allocated for the National Cancer Institute, the report demanded another $220 million immediately to initiate the programme and then an additional $150 million a year, reaching $1 billion by 1976.

Central to this endeavour was a proposal to create an organisation called the National Cancer Authority to manage the cancer quest: its director would be appointed by the President, and its budget agreed directly. The idea of this new institution was to cut through the bureaucratic tangle of the National Cancer Institute, which was governed by the National Institutes of Health, and to secure the funds for clinical research that Mary Lasker and her friends thought appropriate. Of course, these were only recommendations. The laws to implement them would have to be made in Congress and Senate during the following twelve months.

Just two weeks after the report's launch, the film *Love Story* was released with the opening lines, 'What can you say about a 24-year-old girl who died?' Telling the story of her illness, which appears to be cancer, it won rave reviews, filled cinemas and contributed to a public mood that was certainly receptive to the campaign of Lasker and her friends.

While Republican members of the panel lobbied President Nixon's aides, Lasker and Schmidt went to Elmer Bobst to suggest that the President mention the cancer initiative in the State of the Union address in January. Inside the White House, there was already some concern that the Cancer Program was building political capital for Senator Teddy Kennedy, who had taken Yarborough's place as the champion of the bill. As Kennedy might be the Democratic presidential contender in 1972, Nixon, who had been elected in 1968, was keen to pre-empt him. So, in front of the joint session of Congress, on 22 January 1971, the President announced an extra $100 million for cancer research in his State of the Union address – which he later told Lasker was the result of Bobst's lobbying. 'The time has come in America,' said Nixon, 'when the same kind of concentrated effort that split the atom and took man to the moon should be turned toward conquering this dread disease. Let us make a total national commitment to achieve this goal.'

However, although these broad commitments were announced, there was still no legislation to implement them. Mary Lasker still had much to battle for.

Late one evening, forty weeks after his diagnosis, Dad telephoned me. Because of the hour, at first I feared that something was wrong, but then I realised he was just back to his old tricks, staying up long into the night. We made arrangements for later in the week: I was going to accompany him to a lunch of the society of printers and designers, for whom he had been printing a keepsake.

On the morning of the day that we were supposed to meet, I had unearthed a video of Nixon's State of the Union address. The President walks through the crowded, cheering House towards the podium, then delivers his speech. In one sense, it seemed so much part of history. At the same time, the filigrees of hope that Nixon represented had invaded my own world. For, as he was being cheered, the idea of cancer being a curable disease, as liable as the moon to surrender to human endeavour, was being placed in the centre of the public imagination.

Dad seemed positively youthful at the lunch. He was carrying hundreds of copies of the keepsake that he had spent so long printing. But in the taxi on the way there, he decided that he had failed to attain a level of sufficient quality, so he kept them in his briefcase. Although his body was collapsing and there was no real reason for optimism, he felt that there would be plenty of other opportunities to print them more beautifully.

Similarly, Mum and I continued to wish into the void. I understood that the disease was wearing him down, but I was still convinced that some future treatment, some kind of medical intervention, would beat it. My friends, too, seemed to be infected with this kind of optimism, for when I described Dad's illness, a common-enough response was to say 'Maybe there will be a cure soon.'

After the speaker at the lunch, Dad proved his vitality by asking the first question. Then he wished his friends goodbye.

I put him in a taxi as he rushed off to see an exhibition at Tate Britain; he was filling every available minute until the train home.

❧

The National Cancer Act – as it would eventually be named – required the ratification of both Houses and the President to become law. Yet in the weeks following Nixon's State of the Union address, the broader scientific community mounted a concerted counter-attack. They were not, of course, resisting the massive infusion of money but were objecting to the establishment of a centralised National Cancer Agency that was separate from the National Institutes of Health. One critic suggested that it would be managed by 'uncritical zealots, by experts in advertising and public relations, and rapacious "empire builders"', referring to Lasker and her friends.

One of the roots of this debate was a fundamental disagreement over the possibility of managing science. Invoking what might be called the Law of Unintended Consequences, the scientific establishment held the view that progress was unpredictable, as great discoveries often happened in unexpected fields and were frequently authored by young, maverick investigators, working in institutions at the peripheries. The history of medicine was replete with examples where scientists had wandered down an apparently aimless research avenue only to stumble on a medically applicable insight. The creation of antibiotic medicine, for example, was initiated by a chance observation of how a mould was killing bacteria in Petri dishes. Similarly, the development of the polio vaccine was made possible only by the fortuitous discovery that the polio virus would reproduce in the brains of monkeys. Indeed, just the year before Nixon's announcement, two brilliant scientists – Howard Temin from the University of Wisconsin and David Baltimore from the Massachusetts Institute of Technology – had discovered the mechanism of an arcane animal cancer virus, which had led to profound insights into the functioning of all genes. Hailed as one of the great biological discoveries of the century, its authors would go on to share a Nobel Prize. At the time, it was also thought that spin-offs of the research would immediately be applied to cancer – though the research had not been envisioned with that purpose. So when Baltimore testified at a congressional hearing, he objected to the establishment of a National Cancer Agency and a targeted plan that would centralise cancer research because 'it will not speed up and may slow down progress and because the American people should not be misled into thinking that a cure for cancer is imminent'.

By contrast, Lasker's friends were impatient. 'The 325,000 patients with cancer who are going to die this year cannot wait,' declared Sidney Farber, 'nor is it necessary, in order to make great progress in the cure of cancer, for us to have the full solution of all problems of basic research.' But during 1971, Lasker's proposals for a NASA-type National Cancer Agency and a meticulously managed plan for cancer research were rejected by Congress and the Senate. Her consolation was that her lobbying had not only safeguarded her achievements of the previous twenty years, but had also increased the budget of the National Cancer Institute to $379 million.

The result was the National Cancer Act, signed on 23 December 1971. 'For this legislation – perhaps more than any legislation I have signed as President of the United States – can mean new hope and comfort in the years ahead for millions of people in the country and around the world,' said Nixon. The Act's main component was a series of regulations re-organising the National Cancer Institute and giving greater powers to its director. Included in the audience of invited guests was Mary Lasker. 'It was a beautiful day in Washington,' Lasker remembered. 'And we didn't know until the very last minute whether he was going to sign it or not, in a big ceremony, but finally he signed it in the dining room of the White House about noon, and there were about 250 people there, many of whom had done their utmost to defeat the bill in one way or another, all taking a lot of credit and drinking coffee and talking to each other.'

However, despite Lasker's success in increasing the federal cancer budget, she had essentially lost her fight to control where the money was spent, and she was disappointed. 'People at the National Institutes of Health are not businessmen,' Lasker despaired in the mid 1970s. 'They're research administrators who are not interested in getting anything accomplished. They don't have any consuming drive to solve anything.'

By 1974, four years after Lasker's panel had been established, policy makers had lost faith that a centrally managed, concerted effort would succeed against a single disease group, and instead subscribed to the belief that science was a broad endeavour in which the insights from one field became the foundations for advances in others. The failure of the moon-shot approach to medical research was exemplified by the Special Virus Cancer Program, which had produced no convincing results in the decade since its foundation. The hoped-for vaccine turned out to be mere speculation. A government study in 1974 concluded that virologists were no nearer to finding either a human cancer virus or a vaccine, despite spending $250 million; some of the reports of success in the previous years had been the result of laboratory contamination or human error: 'There did not, nor does there, exist knowledge to mount such a narrowly targeted program.' The rationale for Building 41 and its supporting institutions was effectively demolished by the report. Moreover, the report stated, the managed and directed programme had been detrimental to the free-thinking and collegiate process of science; rather, a self-sustaining bureaucracy had been established in which research contracts were given to scientists who were part of the 'in group', rather than those who held alternative views.

Despite the organisational setbacks and the failure to discover a vaccine, Lasker continued to search for a cure, her hope undimmed.

*

When I next went home, forty-two weeks after diagnosis, Dad's health had declined. Walking was now difficult, and he had taken to wheeling himself backwards in an old office chair using his good leg and his arms. I was there with my girlfriend Andrea and her daughter, Linnéa. Out of nostalgia as much as teenage entertainment, I decided to teach Linnéa how to set our home address in Dad's lead type. As Dad was himself no longer able to get through the cluttered garage to the type cases, the next day we placed his smallest printing press on the kitchen table. Sitting in his pyjamas, Dad gave instructions and oversaw the procedure. When the printing surface needed to be delicately adjusted, he wielded his scalpel, the pieces of padding paper and his ruler. After some struggle, we printed for the rest of the afternoon. Dad was collapsed on his bed when we left, so exhausted that I wondered if he'd ever wake.

A few days later, the doctor pronounced his neck and shoulders in good health, but was worried by the fact that Dad's painful left hip had now shrunk to half the size of his right.

Wiser than us all, Dad began for the first time to talk about his funeral. Initially, I refused to discuss the arrangements but late one night he became insistent. As a piece of music for entering and leaving the chapel, he said, he would like Beethoven's Serenade for String Trio in D major, Opus 8. He extracted the score from his library, and relived the moment when he had first heard it: forty years before, on moving to Birmingham, he had stood at the back of a recital in the cathedral. It was a good piece of music for funerals, he said, because it had a rapid tempo and was not a dirge. He suggested that a neighbourhood group might be prevailed upon to perform.

That night, sitting across from me in the kitchen, he seemed as strong and as vocal as he had ever been. It seemed inconceivable that we were discussing his death.

&.

Mary Lasker was often asked by friends and colleagues for advice about their own cancer diagnoses and treatments. Having long been close to the Kennedy clan, she was confronted with a particularly poignant case in November 1973, when the 12-year-old son of Senator Edward Kennedy had his leg amputated above the knee to curtail a rare bone cancer. As well as sending notes, good wishes and flowers, she telephoned Edward Senior to encourage further treatment: new combinations of chemotherapy might reduce the risk of recurrence. Kennedy began to research his son's cancer by visiting the Memorial Sloan-Kettering Hospital in New York and by organising a seminar of seven of the leading cancer specialists in his Georgetown home; and when Teddy Junior began an intensive course of chemotherapy at the beginning of February 1974, his father learnt how to give him the required fortnightly injections. Teddy Junior wrote to Mary Lasker, 'Thank you for sending your feelings, notes and thoughts and remembering me in your prayers. The little time it took you to write these notes encouraged me greatly, and now I am just beginning to walk.'

Teddy Junior's cancer and his survival were widely reported, and his father discussed the options and the prognosis in the press. Unlike previous generations who had silently borne their cancers, public figures now talked about the disease. This trend reached new heights shortly after the resignation of Richard Nixon, when in September 1974, the new first lady, Betty Ford, announced that she was herself a breast cancer patient, provoking a wave of public support during which she received 50,000 letters. As one correspondent wrote, 'You have made us love you in a short while.'

Meanwhile, Mary Lasker steadfastly held to her view that a magic bullet might exist, encouraged by the success of chemotherapy treatments such as those offered to Teddy Kennedy Junior and to childhood leukaemia patients. 'Mary Lasker wanted something dramatic to happen, something that went "whammo" against cancer,' said one of her associates.

In 1975, Lasker's gaze alighted upon interferon, a complex and barely understood protein named after its apparent ability to disrupt the life cycle of various viruses, which had been discovered almost twenty years previously. Lasker's aspirations were supported by a single piece of clinical evidence: a Finnish study had revealed, a few years before, that interferon had prolonged the lives of fourteen children with the same rare bone cancer that had afflicted young Teddy Kennedy; yet, unlike chemotherapy drugs, it had few toxic side effects. Studies in mice also showed that interferon arrested cancer. This all-but-mythical elixir was almost impossible to manufacture, however. Only one place in the world, the State Serum Institute in Helsinki, and one man, Kari Cantell, had managed to extract and isolate sufficient quantities from donated human blood for studies in patients. But even he required the blood donations of 70,000 people to produce just a quarter of a gram, hardly sufficient for a handful of patients.

That interferon might cure cancer in humans, Lasker thought, was 'simply thrilling', so thrilling that she turned her considerable energy towards securing enough interferon for a full clinical trial. 'I am perfectly aware of what I try to do and what I am successful at. It would annoy the hell out of most people, because they'd say anybody that had been able to get that much done had too much power,' she said. Initially she sent associates to Helsinki to negotiate with Cantell; she also encouraged her friend Mathilde Krim, the Memorial Sloan-Kettering scientist with whom she had lobbied Senator Yarborough back in 1969, to organise a conference on the possibilities presented by interferon, which was attended by doctors, scientists and pharmaceutical executives. With interest in interferon growing, Lasker sold some of her impressionist paintings to buy $800,000 worth of the drug for a larger clinical trial. Partly as a consequence of Lasker's lobbying, and that of her friends, the American Cancer Society and the National Institutes of Health each then pledged $2 million to pay Cantell to produce a few more spoonfuls that could be tested on patients.

Even before the first small-scale clinical trials had begun in America, an unknown company called Genentech announced in 1977 that they had manufactured a complex human protein by a revolutionary method called 'genetic engineering', thereby giving birth to the biotechnology industry, which promised the mass production of cheap protein-based drugs. Seeing the potential for manufacturing interferon, Mary Lasker began touring companies and venture capitalists, encouraging them to clone the drug. 'Now of course it's going to make some scientists quite rich, and this is very annoying to other scientists, but if it gets products that will prevent the common cold, the flu and shingles, and will certainly treat – we hope – the major cancers, that doesn't seem to be very serious,' said Lasker.

That cancer might succumb to a magic bullet worth billions of dollars encouraged venture capitalists throughout Europe, America and Japan to seek out the best university microbiologists and challenge them to manufacture interferon. One of the many scientists who began chasing the interferon rainbow was a professor of microbiology at the University of Zürich called Charles Weissmann, who co-founded a company called Biogen, in 1978. Shrewdly, Weissmann procured interferon-producing cells from Kari Cantell. Yet even then, and although Genentech had proven the principle of genetic engineering, Weissmann found it challenging to unravel the mechanisms with which human cells produced the drug. Eventually, in December 1979, he succeeded, describing the feeling as the 'utter bliss which comes only rarely in a scientific lifetime'. Within days, Biogen had lodged patents and three weeks later the news broke. Within a few months, interferon had made the front cover of *Time* magazine.

As *Science* magazine declared, this was 'the date on which molecular biology became big business'. Until then, most cancer scientists had been motivated by the urge to advance medical knowledge for the betterment of mankind, funded by government or large charities. While some had sought celebrity – wishing to become as famous as the heart transplant pioneer Christian Barnard – now money became part of the equation.

Although the genetic engineering of interferon promised a cheaper, more abundant supply, it would take some years for Biogen to bring the technique fully into commercial production. In the meantime, the drug manufactured by Cantell from human cells, which Lasker and others had raised millions of dollars to buy, was being tested on patients. Initially, one trial with small numbers of cancer patients in Houston showed that those who took the drug seemed to live longer than those who had not taken the drug. But when larger quantities of the genetically engineered protein were then used in trials in Houston and around the world, they showed that a placebo was just as effective. The earlier positive results from Finland, and those from tests elsewhere with small numbers of patients, were false, the result of experimental error. After all the hype, patients were left with only their hopes and the yellowing press clippings. 'We paid heavily in terms of all this publicity,' one of the trial doctors said. 'The demands on the patients, the disappointments when we didn't have a cure.'

For science as a whole, the interferon crusade demonstrated the unintended consequences of the new commercial pressures on science. While the influx of private money brought some researchers freedom from the government bureaucrats who had previously controlled their budgets, it also divided a community that had once harnessed the scientific method towards the common good. Researchers found themselves signing contracts and confidentiality agreements that constrained them from publishing their work. Money itself skewed the relationships of scientists. Kari Cantell, for instance, never received any money from Biogen, despite supplying them with interferon-producing cells. When asked later what he thought about their behaviour, he commented simply, 'They did not offer, and I did not ask.'

&a.

Eleven months after Dad's surgery, he woke weak and pale one morning and was rushed by ambulance to the Accident and Emergency department of our local hospital. By coincidence, I had been on my way to visit. His previous ward had been in a modern building, close to all the latest technology, but he had now been admitted to a red-brick Victorian sanatorium that had seen better days.

I found him on a bed in the hectic ward with Mum. His left hip seemed to be wasting away, and when he moved, needles of pain shot through his body. When I lifted his leg, however, there was some respite. His skin was white and clammy. A little greasy perhaps, as if colour – and with it life – were draining from his body. I spent hours holding Dad's leg in the air as he waited. When the doctors finally came, all they prescribed were painkillers and a quieter ward.

&a.

Coming fast on the heels of failed campaigns to develop a range of chemotherapies and vaccines for every cancer, interferon's failure to be cancer's magic bullet stripped bare the empty promises of those directing cancer research towards immediate therapeutic ends. Neither the good intentions of philanthropists, nor the actions of governments, nor even the determination to turn a profit, could guarantee a specific scientific outcome. The failure humbled science. Of course, surgery, radiation and chemotherapy were powerful treatments in certain circumstances, but none was as powerful as a polio vaccine, or as immediately effective as penicillin on bacteria. The despair and anger that patients felt, and still feel, at medicine's apparent impotence is in part the result of too many unfulfilled promises.

The abject failure of the 'war on cancer', which had been waged since Nixon's announcement in 1971, was tellingly described by two statisticians, John C. Bailar III and Elaine Smith, in 1986. Reviewing cancer data from the previous thirty years, they demonstrated that 'mortality rates have shown a slow and steady increase over several decades, and there is no evidence of a downward trend'. The primary driver of this 8 per cent rise was lung cancer. Had lung cancer deaths been excluded, then the rates would have shown a 13 per cent decline. Nonetheless, they said, 'The main conclusion we draw is that 35 years of intense effort focused largely on improving treatment must be judged a qualified failure', closing with the words, 'We are losing the war on cancer.'

Mary Lasker had a somewhat different perspective: 'I think that our efforts have been too small, not too big, and what they call the immense amount of money spent for it is peanuts compared to what it should have been. That's my comment on that.' Although she often doubted the managerial abilities of scientific administrators, she had raised vast sums for their coffers. By the mid 1980s, the combined spending of the National Institutes of Health – including the National Cancer Institute – was close to $4.5 billion a year and Lasker was rightly proud. 'If it hadn't been for me,' she said, 'there wouldn't have been any National Institutes of Health as it exists, nor the money available.' And though the schemes that she most favoured failed to produce an immediate cancer cure, they did enormously benefit medicine. The Special

Virus Cancer Program of the late 1960s and early 1970s, for instance, created the foundations for identifying the AIDS virus after the disease emerged in the early 1980s, as well as for studying the genetic basis of cancer. Likewise, interferon became a valuable treatment for some rare cancers such as hairy cell leukaemia and for hepatitis. Today, there is even a resurgence of interest in human cancer viruses, as scientists estimate that about 5 per cent of all cancers are caused by viruses; moreover, a new vaccine is arriving on the market which should protect women from cervical cancer.

Lasker had also contributed greatly to the fields that she had most often disdained: those of unpredictable basic science. By 1980, investigators following their own peculiar interests, unfettered by some grander managerial vision, and publicly funded, had discovered a multitude of ways to manipulate genes by cutting and recombining the long chains of DNA. Although she had often complained about this kind of research, the money that she had raised had assisted significantly its advancement. In 1981, she admitted that had she seen the grant applications of some of these basic scientists she probably would have said, 'I don't understand this … let's give the money to somebody else.' Yet it was these fundamental observations about manipulating genes and the biology of cells that would provide a foundation for the next great leap of cancer science. As she said, 'You just don't know from whence something is going to come.' She died in 1994 at the age of 93, leaving her foundation to continue her work.

❧

When I next saw Dad, a few days after his readmission to hospital, he was lying on his back holding a broadsheet newspaper with two arms. Although he now found books too heavy to hold for long periods, he did not want to be left behind by world events.

When I asked Dad about the progress of his treatment,

he told me that he had told his medical history to the ward's doctors, but no specialist had had the time to diagnose him. This was partly because they were waiting for results of yet more MRI and bone scans to be able to plot the course of his disease, but also because they had too few resources to cope with the demand.

As a family we imagined that Dad would soon undergo some sort of treatment, buoyed up by his experience of the previous year when medicine had saved him. Surely something could now be done? Amid the frantic rhythm of the hospital and Dad's requirements for clean clothes, fresh fruit and entertaining company, we had become as delusional and optimistic as the science policy makers of the 1970s. We had lost sight of the possibility that there might be another scenario, one in which he would die. Instead we began to meet with palliative care nurses and ask them questions about what Dad would need once he had recovered and been discharged. For a while, we became experts in different models of wheelchair, comparing their specifications as if we were trying to purchase a car. Although he found walking difficult, Dad was otherwise in good spirits. And, after the initial crisis, friends had begun to visit and cheer him up.

It was my birthday a week after Dad was pitched back into hospital. Although it was early afternoon when I arrived, Dad was still asleep. The role reversal shocked me: I remembered the nights when I was supposed to be sleeping, and he would feel my bedside light to discover if I had been reading surreptitiously. In the end, he stirred as his grandchildren arrived. Once Dad had lifted himself into a wheelchair and wrapped himself in his dressing gown, I pushed him down the long corridors to the canteen where my sister sat guarding a chocolate fudge birthday cake. My sister's children were running around, excited by the prospect of a birthday party even though the hospital by-laws prohibited candles. As the whole family sang, Dad looked up, his sparkling eyes dancing, his face brimming with joy.

Alternatives:

the backlash against orthodoxy

In the autumn of 1979, Penny Brohn, who lived near Bath in the south-west of England, found a large, painful lump in her left breast. Aged 36 and with three children, she brushed the worst possibilities aside. 'Oh, it can't be cancer,' she thought, 'because everybody told me that tumours were always small and not painful.' Her doctor agreed but suggested a biopsy 'to be on the safe side', just a simple 'quickie' operation. As she was an acupuncturist, she asked to administer her own pain relief, but her doctors refused. So under only local anaesthetic she watched her surgeon's forehead ripple with frown lines and the nurses grow more agitated as they wrestled with her lump. The operation dragged on, and it became something more like a lumpectomy. Bleeding volumes, she found the pain intolerable.

Afterwards, when she was lying in the ward, her doctor told her that it was, in fact, cancer. 'His management of my crisis consisted of a pat on the hand and the assurance that he was very sorry. I didn't feel sorry was worth much,' she wrote; the fear, anger, panic and guilt were 'massive and overwhelming'. To be so uninformed and disempowered was difficult for someone as single-minded as Brohn, but her doctor insisted that her recovery had nothing to do with her own will.

As the days passed, she experienced what she described as an 'existential crisis', questioning who she was, what her life was for and where it was going. Then, although her doctors eventually offered her a mastectomy in order to complete the job that they had begun, she refused. One doctor suggested that she was throwing her life away; another insisted that the decision should be taken out of her hands. 'If the hospital had been dealing a good line in lifetime guarantees along with their wares,' she wrote, 'then I would have been just another grateful customer.' As it was, she discharged herself with a weeping wound, 'a big bundle of sterile dressings and not the faintest idea of what I would do next'.

So begins the story of Penny Brohn – in the years ahead, she would tell and retell this story as the incitement and inspiration for her life's work. Narratives such as Brohn's, heartbreaking tales of determination and survival from courageous patients and maverick doctors, were often used by advocates for the alternative medical movement of the 1970s. Gilded with countercultural, anti-authoritarian ideas, which mirrored the political mood of the time, these heroics gained great currency in the media and were well received by the public. They also formed the evidence upon which the alternative medical movement based its theories, a departure from orthodox medicine's reliance upon the statistically based scientific reports found in the medical journals.

Penny Brohn's story was the foundation of a radical cancer centre that would eventually be endorsed by some of Britain's most established institutions, including the heir to the throne. As a consequence, she became one of the most successful propagators of alternative medical ideas in the world, and emblematic of the movement as a whole.

Although there were many different schools of alternative medicine, ranging from the use of ancient herbs to mind-over-body techniques, its therapists, including Brohn, for the most part subscribed to a similar critique of orthodox medicine. The critique was most eloquently articulated by the defrocked Jesuit priest Ivan Illich in his 1975 book *Medical Nemesis*, in which he complained about the dehumanising machinery of modern hospitals, clinics and health campaigns. He saw the doctor as a 'pathogen alongside resistant strains of bacteria, hospital corridors, poisonous pesticides and badly engineered cars', who caused pain, injury and suffering. In this view of medicine, patients were hapless victims of uncompassionate, patrician doctors who failed to explain diagnoses or treatments properly. Other critics from the alternative movement singled out cancer therapies as being particularly dangerous: chemotherapy was a toxic brew that killed healthy cells as well as cancerous ones; radiation caused cancer as well as treating it; and surgery mutilated as much as healed.

Although extreme, parts of this critique had much merit. The radical mastectomy, for instance, which involved the excision of the complete breast, a chest muscle and various lymph nodes, had been the surgeon's treatment of choice for eighty years. Yet there was much evidence to suggest that the excision of a small lump followed by radiation was as successful for most breast cancers. Dissenting doctors had been trying futilely to persuade the mostly male surgeons of this fact for more than forty years. Similarly, the medical profession's faith in chemotherapy during the 1960s and 1970s had increased the pain and disability of some cancer patients without extending or improving the quality of their lives in the final months. Even hospital architecture, with its harsh lines, cold floors and big desks, mirrored the lack of warmth with which many doctors dealt with patients' feelings.

※

After more than a week on the ward, Dad still hadn't been seen by a cancer specialist. The only medical decision the doctors had taken had been to stop the anti-inflammatory drug that he had been using for six weeks – for, far from helping, we feared that the drug might actually be contributing to his decline. He had more X-rays, and then he was wheeled to a magnetic resonance scanner. The results, a few days in coming, suggested that there were new tumours, one at the base of his spine and others in his leg. It was forty-five weeks after his first diagnosis.

On hearing this, my mind emptied. I searched for something to give me a feeling of control, but, finding none, I became angry at the only institution that seemed to have any, the hospital. Their apparent sluggishness – the fact that they had failed to arrange an appointment with a cancer specialist, or to set a course of treatment – became the focus of my rage. That they had succeeded so brilliantly once before had convinced me that they could triumph once again. Even when I visited Dad over the next few days, I encouraged him to get up and walk because I didn't want his body to atrophy; surely he would be up and about shortly. Feeling betrayed at the doctors' inaction, I found *Medical Nemesis* on Dad's shelves and, reading it, found a kind of solace in its bleakness. Had his doctors honestly told me his prognosis, I would have been deaf to their words. I did not have the heart to believe that Dad was being beaten not by man but by a folly of nature.

❦

A few weeks after her diagnosis, Penny Brohn flew to the Bavarian clinic of Josef Issels, which would become very famous a year later when Bob Marley was treated there in the months preceding his death from cancer. Brohn had chosen Issels because he shared her radical view of the human body, a view that stood in contrast to the ideas of orthodox doctors who believed, in the spirit of Rudolf Virchow, that her disease was located at a specific site and was due to the malfunctioning of a particular group of cells. 'The most significant feeling I had,' she thought, 'was that my cancer involved the whole of me, not just a bumpy bit on the left side', an idea that she had picked up while studying acupuncture in Hong Kong a few years before.

Disease was not only physical, she believed, but the manifestation of the collapse of the mind and the spirit: 'I knew that my cancer was an accumulation of un-discharged grief, pent-up guilt and layer upon layer of fear' – an echo, perhaps, of Galen's melancholic humour. So, even before the course of treatment had begun, she dealt with the psychodramas that she thought were affecting her prognosis by confronting her husband on the recriminating gridlock of their marriage. Apparently, the result was a discussion of great warmth: 'this was our first tentative offering of unconditional love, and it felt wonderful'. The reconciliation was centrally important, she believed, to her own eventual good health. She told this story many times, in the years to come, as the cornerstone of her own dramatic story of recovery. 'I am one of the many people who say they are glad they had cancer ... [because of] the indescribable sweetness and joy that came from that night.'

The guiding idea of Issels's clinic, which Brohn enthusiastically embraced, was that it was possible to turn the whole body against cancer. On the one hand, she refused all 'poisons' such as coffee, tea, cigarettes, preservatives, colouring and artificial flavours, and reduced her intake of animal proteins; on the other, she ate raw food, salads, fruits and grains. She pursued this course with such conviction that she never faltered for a cup of coffee or a mouthful of chocolate. Paradoxically, another element of the detoxification regime was regular coffee enemas – a popular element of alternative cancer medicine since the 1950s when a New York doctor called Max Gerson had first recommended them to his patients, believing that the caffeine stimulated the liver to flush out toxins. Though messy and difficult to self-administer, they were promoted by a steady stream of apparent beneficiaries. Brohn was initially sceptical, but 'I mastered them perfectly well and, much against my will, was forced to admit that I felt better for them.' As well as detoxification, Issels attempted to stimulate Brohn's immune system, prescribing a range of dietary supplements, vitamins and homoeopathic remedies.

The popularity of supplements within the alternative movement had much to do with the relentless campaign of Linus Pauling. Although by the 1970s he was in his seventies, he had spent much of the decade berating chat-show hosts and being interviewed for magazines in order to promote the idea that mega-doses of vitamin C 'may turn out to be the most effective and most important substance in the control of cancer', reducing the rates of incidence and mortality by 75 per cent. He brought to the cancer debate an unassailable scientific reputation as the only man to have received two unshared Nobel Prizes – one for chemistry, in recognition of his description of how atoms bond together, and the other for peace as a result of his anti-nuclear campaigning.

In the year that Penny Brohn's cancer was diagnosed, Pauling published his book *Cancer and Vitamin C*, which featured a series of case histories of cancer patients, including a 43-year-old Scottish lorry driver who had, apparently, been cured of lymphatic cancer by taking large doses of vitamin C. More mainstream cancer doctors complained that a handful of good stories did not demonstrate a principle, and were incensed by Pauling's media performances. What was required, they argued, was a comparison between a set of patients who took vitamin C and a similar set who did not. When one such trial showed that vitamin C was of little use, Pauling vigorously contested its methods and sued the researchers, painting himself as the David against the Goliath of the established institutions. The simmering, acrimonious dispute did little, however, to resolve the issue of whether vitamin C had any benefit. But Pauling's reputation had certainly helped to shed doubt on the methods of the orthodox medical community and to bolster the growing alternative health movement.

For nine weeks, Brohn followed Issels's regimen, trying some therapies that she found a little esoteric, such as having her blood oxygenated and fevers induced. She also nurtured her emotional well-being, writing messages of positive reinforcement and repeating them like mantras. 'It's a bugger, it's a bugger, it's a bugger,' she screamed against the tumour into the cold air of the Bavarian hills. As she grew stronger, she became determined to establish a place in England where cancer patients could find similar support, advice and alternative treatments; albeit with a slightly less dogmatic regimen.

❧

After days of waiting in his hospital bed, Dad was finally given an appointment with the specialist. He lifted himself into a wheelchair, was pushed to a bus, and then driven to another building, a few miles from his ward. For most of the afternoon, he waited uncomfortably, ignored by the nurses and doctors. When the consultant eventually saw him in the early evening, Dad's paperwork had been mislaid. In any case, the doctor demanded a bone scan before he could chart the course ahead. Mum and Helen, Dad's sister, had waited with him; I was in London. They were angry. For my part, I felt he was being neglected when there must have been something – surgery, radiation, chemotherapy, interferon or something, I knew not precisely what – that could be done.

Late at night, Mum and I talked 'strategies'. Mum was exhausted, having spent so many long hours in the hospital and being too anxious to eat. She always carried a dog-eared folder stuffed with the scratched-out notes about, and chronologies of, Dad's illness. Neither of us talked about the prospect that he might die; rather, we concentrated on the nitty-gritty reality over which we felt we had some power. We wanted Dad to be treated, and then to come home, because we thought that away from the bustle and noise of the ward, and with some round-the-clock emotional support, he would recover more quickly. Although we admired medicine, we too had been influenced by the beliefs and critiques of some parts of the alternative health movement.

So we tried to work out what was necessary, in terms of equipment and personnel, to have him at home. And we talked about how aggressive we should be with the hospital. When I told Dad that I thought we should tackle the hospital management, he demanded that no cross words be spoken. He was quietly accepting; nothing was going to ruin his equanimity. As if he had decided not to cause anguish for the family, he determinedly smiled throughout.

On my next visit, Dad was sitting on the edge of the bed. At last he had persuaded doctors to increase the level of morphine to reduce his pain, though this affected his muscular control. His hands shook as he held a glass of water. Moments later, the water spilled all over his pyjamas. Drying him off, we both knew the other saw the accident as an omen. His eyes filled with tears. I told him he was a great father. He replied, 'We just seemed to hit it off.' Neither of us felt comfortable with my holding his hand, and when I told him how much I wished he were well, the words sounded utterly banal.

❧

In the autumn of 1980, Penny Brohn began to recruit cancer patients, from church groups and through friends, who were searching for therapeutic alternatives. In October that year, she welcomed them to a semi-detached house in the suburbs of Bristol, for the first series of advice sessions. Brohn's collaborator and co-founder was Pat Pilkington, a vicar's wife who had previously run a spiritual healing group from the premises and added a determination rooted in her deeply held Christian beliefs to Brohn's passion.

The Bristol Cancer Help Centre was almost unique in the world of alternative therapy insofar as it offered a range of alternative approaches and asked the patients to choose which suited them; most other non-orthodox approaches, including Issels's clinic, dogmatically promoted a single vision. Within a few years, the weekly ad hoc advice session had become a more formalised two-day course. The centre did not advertise, but patients heard about it through friends and alumni, and travelled hundreds of miles for advice and support. Often they were desperate, having reached the limits of what orthodox medicine had to offer. Like Brohn, they were also often angry because the modus operandi of many in the medical profession was brusque and abrupt, lacking in a certain compassion. 'But they arrive at this ordinary house, with pictures on the wall and carpets on the floor,' said Pilkington, 'and all of us looking like normal human beings. No uniforms of any sort. And they are received with love. And that is the thing that distinguishes us: we are voluntary, we all love.'

In the first session of each course, Brohn told the story of her fight against cancer. With a winning smile, she jauntily described her arguments with doctors, her journey to Issels's clinic and her own recovery. As she laced her systematic lessons with self-deprecation, she invited other patients to follow her footsteps. 'Inspire yourself with the thought that there are doctors and clinics all over the world making wonderful claims for these holistic methods,' she wrote – even though alternative practitioners were very much outside the margins of accepted medical practice. The watchwords of this ascetic therapy were discipline, vigour and self-denial.

Mental and spiritual well-being were important elements of the courses too, so patients received counselling – to determine what kind of trauma had caused their disease – and underwent a session of spiritual 'healing' in which the healer would lay on hands, in order to martial forces to fight the cancer. Some patients said that during this experience they felt as if another force had entered their body. Many of the less-religious patients, of which there were quite a few, saw it as a form of meditation.

Another part of the course was led by the third member of the team, a retired physician called Alec Forbes who gave the enterprise a certain medical authority. Rake-thin and toweringly tall, his demeanour was of a rather passionate schoolteacher bringing discipline into the lives of his patients. In one of the centre's pamphlets, he stated that 'it is a fact that people who resist their cancer actively have a much better outcome than those who are apathetic about it'. As well as prescribing a series of vitamin supplements, coffee enemas and various 'alternative' cancer drugs, Forbes dogmatically advocated the Bristol diet, modelled on the one that Brohn had eaten in Bavaria. Every participant was instructed to eat raw fruit and vegetables, to drink many glasses of carrot juice each day, and to be entirely vegan. A typical lunch consisted of fresh carrot juice; a salad of beetroot, courgette, lettuce, bean sprouts, carrots and celery; and orange and banana 'surprise'. The diet required unswerving dedication, constant juicing, specialised sourcing and new recipes. The houses of those patients who adhered to it smelt of carrots, and their skins turned slightly orange. So tough were the demands that about a third of those who attended the courses failed to follow any of the programme when they returned home, and only half subscribed with any degree of commitment. Some of these found it difficult to escape the feeling that they had failed and might suffer the consequences. 'The people who come here and do well,' remarked Pilkington, 'are the people that are committed.'

One other technique taught at Bristol was 'visualisation', as pioneered by the husband-and-wife team Carl and Stephanie Simonton at their clinic in Fort Worth, Texas. Their book, *Getting Well Again*, first published in 1978, was a best-seller and contained the emblematic story of a 61-year-old man who was dying of a cancer of the jaw so severe the patient found it difficult to swallow his own saliva. Carl Simonton instructed him to set aside three 15-minute periods each day, during which he was to relax. Throughout these sessions, the Simontons wrote, 'Carl asked him to picture his treatment, radiation therapy, as consisting of millions of tiny bullets of energy that would hit the cells, both normal and cancerous, in their path.' As cancer cells exploded, the patient was to think of his white cells engulfing the tumour, and of its decreasing in size. 'What happened was beyond any of Carl's previous experience,' they declared. Within two months, the patient's cancer had entirely disappeared.

At the Bristol Centre, patients were taken through this technique and many others, and in general they were enthusiastic. Month by month, the word spread.

❧

Mum found a lump in her breast in the late summer of 1982. Scared and a little ashamed, she shared her trauma with only her sister and her sister-in-law, Helen, a fellow doctor. Not wanting to worry anyone, she didn't even tell her mother she was going into hospital. Aged just 51, she wondered if she would ever see her children grow into adults – I was 14, my sister 17. But she was a doctor and read the journals, and she and her surgeon decided that although the radical mastectomy would have been the normal approach, a lumpectomy would be sufficient. She was so blasé about her operation that her cancer scare has left hardly any traces in my memory, except for the image of a bottle containing the dregs of her blood swinging beneath her hospital bed. When she was discharged from hospital, she sought out the Bristol Cancer Help Centre for support, because she had heard about it on the radio.

They sent her a collection of eight brightly coloured leaflets written by Alec Forbes and Penny Brohn, each one about a different subject, from diet to coffee enemas. Mum warmed to their mantras, such as, 'Positive action is key, never give up', and she accepted that some of these strategies might improve her quality of life, and that counselling, a service not offered by her conventional doctors, might be useful for others. But the more she read, the more the leaflets unsettled her, particularly because of what she regarded as the promises of false hope. 'Do the therapies work?' asked one leaflet. 'If they are followed completely and persistently,' it continued, 'they can and do save life.'

Her greatest objection was that they were promoting laetrile, an extract of apricot kernels, whose most famous adherent in the months leading up to his death from cancer had been the Hollywood icon Steve McQueen. The drug had been the subject of a long, heated battle, and the most recent scientific evidence showed not only that laetrile was of no benefit, but also that it could cause harm. Despite this, Penny Brohn promoted the drug in these leaflets and, later, in various books. Mum also found the dogmatism of the leaflets disturbing, because they gave the impression that those sufferers who did not follow the rigid regimen were welcoming doom.

❧

Though my mother never made the journey to the Bristol Cancer Help Centre, many others did. As its fame rose steadily, various members of the orthodox medical establishment criticised the centre's approach – but Penny Brohn and Pat Pilkington's passion and determination, and their shrewd encouragement of the media, meant that the centre continued to grow. Soon they began to look for new, larger premises.

The Centre's public exposure increased further in March 1983, when the BBC broadcast a documentary series called *A Gentle Way With Cancer?*. Studiously measured, the six-part series concentrated on meditation, counselling, visualisation and spiritual healing, and avoided controversy by repeatedly emphasising that the therapies were complementing rather than replacing orthodox medicine. Nonetheless, the BBC appeared to be supporting the new approach, such that in the weeks before its broadcast various doctors attempted unsuccessfully to persuade the broadcaster that the series ought not to be transmitted.

In June that year, the Bristol Approach found even greater endorsement when the Prince of Wales opened the new building, a former nunnery. He told the crowds that just because treatments 'at physical, emotional and spiritual levels cannot be proved in a clinical laboratory to have a value to patients, does not mean [they are] completely worthless or harmful'. Though Charles had a reputation for championing eccentric causes, on this occasion he was reflecting the public mood. A few weeks later, even the editorial pages of *The Times* joined the fray, stating that 'in cancer as in most other serious conditions, science has not earned the right to demand absolute conviction from patients', and praised the Bristol Centre.

Few if any non-orthodox medical centres anywhere in the world had garnered so much authority. By contrast, many American practitioners had been forced to work out of a cluster of clinics in Tijuana, Mexico, because during the 1970s there had been a concerted campaign by the Food and Drugs Administration to arrest laetrile salesmen and force other therapists out of business so that only registered doctors could give health advice. But although Penny Brohn and Pat Pilkington were not prevented from offering such help, the medical profession had their knives out.

❦

When the doctors finally found time and had amassed sufficient information to see my father, two weeks after admission, they recommended one final dose of radiation. As we waited in the radiation suite, he sat reading in his wheelchair. He had always said he was a slow reader, but that day he read huge chunks, sucking up information.

When they eventually wheeled him off, the consultant ushered Mum and me into an office. He pulled magnetic resonance images of Dad, which had been taken a few days earlier, out of an envelope and mounted them on a light box. There were more than a dozen sections through the middle of the body, grey swirling masses that looked more like weather formations than body parts. The socket in the joint of Dad's hip had all but collapsed. Not only would walking therefore increase his pain, but there was now the terrible risk that his thigh bone, his femur, might break through his hip and lodge fatally in his abdomen. So while this burst of radiation might reduce his pain, it would not make Dad mobile again. When we asked how long Dad had to live, the doctor said maybe months, maybe weeks.

As we walked away, Mum became concerned that any medical intervention might be detrimental to my father's quality of life in his final days. She feared that the radiation, rather than helping his pain, might make him more uncomfortable and his last days more unbearable, pushing him closer to death. It was as if all the promises, all the hopes that had been conjured up in the previous year, were for nothing. Medicine's sophisticated models of human biology were worthless when faced with dying Dad. Despite being a doctor herself, she now became nervously uncertain as to whether medicine had any benefit to offer him. So she turned around and began to hurry back towards the consultant.

Eventually, when we tracked him down, Mum asked him to justify his decision. I had never seen Mum's steel until she stood there demanding, questioning and arguing. Though he seemed a little irritated to be doubted, the consultant told her that recent studies had shown that although a bolt of radiation was unlikely to slow greatly the progression of the disease, it would reduce pain. He offered to dig out the papers that he was referring to. But Mum's resolve had withered; it seemed that the decision was based on firm grounds.

In the ambulance on the way back to his ward, Dad's unanswered question was, 'Does the treatment mean I'll be able to walk again?'

§.

In 1986, Penny Brohn and Pat Pilkington invited a group of scientists to the Bristol Cancer Help Centre to discuss the possibility of doing a scientific study that they hoped would prove the success of the Bristol Approach in treating cancer patients.

Sir Walter Bodmer, the director general of Britain's largest cancer charity, the Imperial Cancer Research Fund (ICRF), and a renowned statistician, made the journey. As did Professor Tim McElwain, from the Institute of Cancer Research in London – even though he had been one of the Bristol Centre's most trenchant critics. The week before Prince Charles had visited the centre, for instance, McElwain had complained to *The Times* that 'royalty should not be endorsing bogus techniques'. He strongly disagreed with the claims that the hotchpotch of medicines, diets and supplements could extend the lives of patients, stating in a television discussion of the centre, 'I have seen no evidence that it works.'

McElwain was not, however, a blinkered, uncompassionate doctor of the old school, and he shared Brohn and Pilkington's view of the way that some doctors treated patients. 'I think [the Bristol Centre] highlights ... our failure as doctors particularly in our relationship with our patients,' he said in the same television discussion. 'This recurrent theme that patients are not involved in their own treatment, that they are improperly informed, that not enough time is taken with them and that there is often a lack of respect for them, by some doctors, though by no means all, is the thing that is important.' To this end, in 1984, he had become the vice-chair of the newly formed British Association of Cancer United Patients (BACUP), which was to provide advice and emotional support to patients. The need was clearly there, as during the first year BACUP received 30,000 phone calls.

Shortly after the visit of Bodmer and McElwain, the Imperial Cancer Research Fund agreed to pay for a small study. 'This means that in a few years' time,' trilled Penny Brohn when the study was underway, 'we should be able to produce the facts and the figures to support what we believe to be true, that time spent at Bristol can have a profound effect on the performance and survival of cancer patients.'

The research study was led by Claire Chilvers, a professor of epidemiology at the Institute of Cancer Research, with McElwain supplying the clinical expertise. Initially they had hoped to randomly allocate women who arrived at Bristol into two groups: those receiving the Bristol Programme and those receiving nothing. But Pilkington and Brohn thought it was unethical to refuse treatment to some patients; and since they had sought out Bristol they would be unlikely to forgo the treatment once they had arrived. So McElwain and Chilvers decided to follow a group of patients from Bristol and compare them to case histories of patients drawn from the files of two district hospitals.

Women arriving at Bristol during the summer of 1986 were each handed a detailed questionnaire about their states of mind, the extent to which they followed the Bristol Programme and what kind of psychological benefit they found. Each year, these women answered the questions again.

As the research was being conducted, Penny Brohn had a recurrence of her breast cancer. 'She was struggling with feeling guilty about being ill again,' remembers Michael Wetzler, the doctor at the Bristol Centre. 'She should have beaten it. Because she believed these ways beat it. So she thought she must have been doing something wrong. Could she find it inside, and get it right?' Reluctantly she underwent surgery, and began taking a drug called tamoxifen, which was supposed to reduce the risk of the cancer returning. A measure of her unease in resorting to more conventional approaches was that in the two books she published in 1986 and 1987, one outlining her personal struggle and the other describing the Bristol Approach, she never mentioned the drug.

On Wednesday 5 September 1990, the media descended on the offices of the Imperial Cancer Research Fund, in London, to hear the results of the study carried out on the Bristol Cancer Help Centre. For the first time, the combined treatments of diet, meditation, healing and counselling had been put to the test by the orthodox medical establishment. In a room bristling with television cameras and newspaper journalists, Professor Tim McElwain took the podium. As one newspaper reported, he was 'bald, sleek, fat and happy with his professional institute tie, striped blue shirt and blue suit'. Professor Claire Chilvers was also in a dark suit, her hair restrained by tortoiseshell slides. In contrast, crowded towards the other end of the podium were Penny Brohn in a polka-dot suit, her hair trailing down her back, and the doctor of the Bristol Centre, Michael Wetzler, dressed in a linen suit. As the Bristol Cancer Help Centre faced the orthodox establishment, they seemed to come from different worlds.

The journalists were handed a copy of the report to be published in *The Lancet* the next day, which stated, 'These results show that women with breast cancer attending the Bristol Cancer Help Centre fare worse than those receiving conventional treatment only.' Having followed 334 women who had attended the centre, the researchers declared that attendees were almost twice as likely to relapse compared with those undergoing more conventional treatments. From the podium, Professor Chilvers suggested that 'there might be some element of the Bristol regime that does harm. The Bristol Centre is known for its diet.'

The following day the *Guardian* ran the story on its front page with the headline 'DOUBLE RISK AT CANCER UNIT'. *The Sun* was typically tabloid: 'DANGER IN A VEGGIE CURE FOR CANCER: MORE VICTIMS DIE AT PRINCE'S CENTRE'. During the press conference, Penny Brohn was in some anguish: it was as if the scientists and the press were attacking her child. Desperately she attempted to defend the role of diet in treating cancer, while McElwain rolled his eyes and sighed. He emphasised that there was not 'one jot, one tittle' of evidence for such a view. He also said, 'I would no longer be able to tell my patients that going to Bristol would do them no harm.' In the end, Brohn was forced to retreat, saying it was 'impossible to imagine how any of these things could be doing anybody any harm'. But McElwain pointed out that people spending £600 to attend the centre for a week expected not only to feel better but to live longer. That evening, the story reached the TV news bulletins.

In the following weeks, bookings at the Bristol Centre began to decline. Charitable trusts began to cut their contributions. Various staff members were made redundant. But soon the letter pages of *The Lancet* began to fill with scientific critiques of the study, citing 'possible weakness in the trial design and the interpretation of the statistical analysis'. Various correspondents suggested that Bristol patients might differ in some way from those cases drawn from hospital archives, pointing out that when like is not compared to like it is easy to create errors of interpretation. Beneath the cold, bare scientific language of those letters was anger. And eventually it was shown that the cancer of Bristol patients was usually more advanced than that of those to whom they had been compared in the hospital archives, because going to Bristol was for many a last resort. They were therefore much more likely to die.

Two months after the press conference, Tim McElwain and Claire Chilvers responded to their critics in *The Lancet*: 'We regret that our paper has created the widespread impression that the Bristol Cancer Help Centre regimen directly caused the differences that we observed in recurrence and survival. This was never stated. In our view it is much more likely that the difference could be explained by increased severity of disease in Bristol Cancer Help Centre attenders.'

In November 1990, Tim McElwain committed suicide. Though plagued with depressions throughout his life, many felt the strain of the Bristol episode had contributed to his final decision.

In 1991, Penny Brohn developed secondary bone tumours. After radiation and more surgery, she died in February 1999, aged 55.

The conflict over the Bristol study was paralleled in many of the other debates about alternative therapies, for there was little evidence, apart from inspiring personal stories, that vitamin C, extracts of apricot kernel, mistletoe, hydrazine sulphate, 'antineoplastons' or any of the alternative therapies prolonged the lives of cancer patients. At the same time, the medical establishment did little to enhance its own reputation by these angry campaigns. There was a hollow ring to its intemperate attacks against alternative practitioners, because they often came from the same doctors who, just a few years before, had promised cures that had then failed to materialise. Without these perfect solutions, patients had begun to search for their own, and they often found solace and compassion offered only by those outside the mainstream. As a consequence, throughout the 1980s the public mood and the market had shifted subtly towards other approaches; soon the medical establishment would be following.

≈

Two weeks after he was readmitted to hospital, Dad's stay seemed to be becoming just a normal part of family life. Jessica, his almost 4-year-old granddaughter, would visit and run around the wards, as if there was nothing unusual about lines of beds filled with immobile old men.

One day, I pushed Dad through the hospital corridors to a corner of sunlight at the top of some hospital steps. Jessica skipped along beside us. I tucked his blanket around his legs and we stared out at the patch of grass outside the hospital. He reached over and tried to squeeze Jessica's nose. She shrieked and ran off into the light. We waited in silence: it was uncomfortable to hold a conversation there, he being lower than I, and with nurses and porters constantly stepping around us. But we were also lost for words.

I pushed him back to the ward. Jessica made a playhouse out of a walking frame with a coat draped over it. Dad winced trying to move himself back to bed, then asked for the walking frame. She was disappointed that her game was over.

&

The Bristol Cancer Help Centre remains in the tranquil, beautiful former nunnery that was opened by Prince Charles. It still offers week-long courses to cancer patients and their families, during which they are taught about a variety of approaches, from healing to visualisation. But while it still serves a vegan lunch, in many other respects it is a different institution to the one of the early 1980s. Patients are no longer encouraged to follow the diet dogmatically; laetrile and high doses of vitamin C are no longer suggested; and there is never any suggestion that orthodox medical treatments should be avoided. In fact, the Bristol Centre has travelled away from these more controversial treatments towards a softer model of palliative care, of support and counselling that has gained the respect and approval of many of the authorities that govern British medicine. Health professionals now seek out its courses. And for many patients the experience is both life-affirming and useful. The Bristol Centre is, therefore, emblematic of the journey, during the last two decades, that many complementary practitioners have undergone, now mostly offering their services as an adjunct rather than an alternative to orthodox medicine.

In equal measure, orthodox medicine has also changed as a result of the growing vociferousness of patients and the alternative health movement of the 1970s and 1980s. At the same time, the hospice movement, which began in Britain in the late 1960s and was transferred to America a few years later, bequeathed to established medicine insights into caring for patients in the last moments of their life.

Walk into most cancer hospitals in the western world these days, and these softer aspects of medicine are in the foreground. Waiting rooms now have comfortable chairs, pictures on walls and a homely atmosphere; most doctors no longer sit behind big wooden desks; and medical schools now teach 'people skills'. Palliative and supportive care, including those methods taught and practised at Bristol, is now seen to be central to patient care. Indeed, many of the courses at the Bristol Cancer Help Centre are for health professionals. Even old players in the cancer establishment have embraced these complementary approaches: the Memorial Sloan-Kettering Hospital placed a full-page advert in the *New York Times* in 1999, which featured a smiling middle-aged woman, wearing a cheerful bandana to hide her hair loss, over the strap line 'My fight against cancer includes chemotherapy, Swedish massage and relaxing to the muffled rhythms of Tibetan drums.' The advert announced Sloan-Kettering's new Integrative Medicine Centre.

Because the battle lines between the orthodox and the complementary camps have become blurred, there has been much greater enthusiasm for rigorously assessing complementary medicine. Many universities around the world now have professors of the subject, and in America the Office of Cancer Complementary and Alternative Medicine now spends more than $129 million annually investigating non-orthodox treatments. Yet, so far, the findings are very equivocal.

Techniques such as acupuncture and visualisation do seem, in some cases, to improve the quality of life of patients – ideas that would have been fiercely contested by the quack-busters of old. Treatments that are intended to prolong life, by contrast, have not fared well under scrutiny. Equally, there is no evidence to suggest that sad, angry or depressed people are more likely to suffer from the disease. Indeed, one recent study suggested that women under stress are less likely to develop breast cancer than their more relaxed counterparts.

As one doctor, who was part of the quack-busting drive of the 1980s, told me, 'We no longer think that we have the monopoly on wisdom.'

≫

For a few days, the single radiation dose seemed to make a small difference, but then Dad continued to slide. There were no more illusions, no more sprinklings of hope. The mindset had changed, and suddenly neither the doctors nor my parents were talking about treatment. Now it was all about 'making things comfortable'.

The fatalism calmed my anger. In the panic of a few weeks earlier, every moment of inaction had seemed to be a missed opportunity, as if Dad's life were slipping cell by cell through our fingers. But now nothing more could be done. We had been slow, perhaps, to give in to this inevitability; the doctors had known long before. Their inaction had nothing to do with hard-heartedness but was their genuine apprecia-tion of the limits of their own discipline.

Even though mostly I could generally accept the prospect of his death, there were moments when I still raged against our powerlessness, when I truly appreciated Ivan Illich's ideas about the dehumanising systems of modern medicine and I had the urge to search for any way – however esoteric

– to forestall Dad's departure from us. But slowly, the grim biological reality of the disease became more deeply rooted in my mind. The failure of medicine was not the fault of the doctors.

Dad was dying as a consequence of nature itself.

Genes:

the search for the cancer code

FORTY-FOUR WEEKS AFTER DIAGNOSIS. I rearranged the blanket on his legs, shifted the coat across his shoulders. I touched the body that enclosed his insurrection. During those days in Selly Oak Hospital, as I helped him into new sets of pyjamas, pushed him to the toilet, and brought a water bottle to his lips, I had a visceral appreciation of his body as never before, like a parent scrutinising the body of their child. The crude intensity of touching Dad, after years of only talking, forced me to understand that I was the reflection of his flesh, through the distorting mirror of time. I realised anew that he had bequeathed to me his slightly hunched shoulders, his wiry, dark hair, the blood vessel that ran across the back of his hands, and the squint of his nose.

As Dad became sicker, he asked for a laptop to capture his memories. I brought one in, and showed him how to use it. But he barely touched it, unable to muster the energy perhaps, or to commit himself to record his final words. Instead, I sat on the edge of the bed and talked about his family. And along the way we talked about the diseases that had killed them. Dad's father, an engineer who was pictured in one of the family photograph albums building the Aswan

Dam, had died of colon cancer aged 84 – having survived prostate cancer the decade before. Within eighteen months of his death, Dad's mother died of rectal cancer.

With Dad ill, I wondered if he had passed on a cancerous predisposition to me, or to my sister. Insistently, Dad asked about whether his genes had anything to do with his cancer.

❦

In the mid 1970s, Robert Weinberg, an associate professor at the Massachusetts Institute of Technology, was asking similar questions. At the time there was much circumstantial evidence, from studying animal cancers and cells in Petri dishes, to suggest that genes drove human cancers. There was also a rare childhood cancer of the eye, which ran in families, indicating that genes were active in its triggering. Yet no such gene could be categorically identified in either the parents or the patients, because the existing experimental techniques were so rudimentary; nor could the chain of events which led to cancer be clearly described in terms of the genes of a human cell.

Nonetheless, Weinberg hoped to turn the theory into fact, an interest that stretched beyond human inheritance. 'We had relatively little interest in curing cancer or helping the human condition,' he wrote about his part of the scientific community. 'Many of us had never seen cancer up close and been moved by its pain and suffering. We had jumped into the game because it was intellectually challenging. We enjoyed trying to puzzle out Mother Nature.'

The problem was that genes exist in an intangible world where distances are measured in billionths of a metre, where assemblages of atoms are held together by clouds of electromagnetic forces. It had been known for decades that genes were simply discrete sections of strands of deoxyribonucleic acid (DNA), the diameter of which was so thin that one male cell contained nearly two metres of it. In a human cell, this length of DNA was cut into forty-six irregular portions, making the twenty-three pairs of chromosomes. Yet because DNA was so small, its iconic twisting double-helix structure had never been seen through a microscope. Nor could it be physically manipulated by the human hand, nor anything that was directly in our control. There were no experimental techniques, therefore, to demonstrate Weinberg's fundamental hypothesis that genes were the motors of human cancer. Instead he was forced to concentrate on formulating questions that he *could* answer – in the hope that these spots of evidence might build up to a broader picture.

Like most molecular biologists, he was searching for insights not only from human genes; inside bacteria, animals and even viruses there existed genes that had the same structure and often behaved in similar ways. Already a few months before, researchers in his laboratory had shown that it was possible, albeit with great difficulty, to take genes from viruses and splice them into the DNA of mouse cells, in a new process called *transfection*.

In February 1978, Weinberg was walking to work, crossing the Longfellow Bridge that spans the Charles River in Boston, ruminating about this tentative new technique. Tramping through the snow-covered landscape, he had an idea: perhaps it would be possible to use transfection to insert genes from cancerous cells into healthy ones, a bit like taking a mechanical part from one machine and placing it in another to test its function. The brilliance of the notion was that, were it to work, it would clearly and simply demonstrate that a gene had caused a cancer. But really Weinberg was reaching beyond the limits of his grasp: it was as if he intended, with finger-crossing optimism, to throw a collection of car parts into a breakers' yard in the hope that one would reinvigorate one of the many cars. Other researchers would have dismissed the idea as too risky and speculative, because, in fact, transfection did not isolate a single gene but took every gene from a particular group of malignant cells and mixed them with millions of other healthy cells in the desperate hope that one cancer gene would enter a healthy cell and spark malignancy. Nonetheless, 'it was an epiphany, a moment of great excitement,' wrote Weinberg later. And needing to make his reputation, as he had only recently secured tenure by what he described as the 'skin of my arse', he was willing to gamble his lab's resources in the hope of making a genuine, world-changing discovery.

However, he did not make the idea work himself. Indeed, his science bore little resemblance to the lonely pursuit of progress mythologised in the lives of people such as Marie Curie. He did not work at a lab bench, and refused to hold pipettes, lay out arrays of test tubes or peer down micro-scopes, always claiming to be too clumsy. Rather his focus was on being a scientific impresario, guiding his small team, including a handful of junior researchers, towards useful and interesting discoveries. Like some kind of Hollywood Golden-Age dealmaker, his job was to manage the stars (his researchers), come up with bankable ideas, make them happen and sell them to the public, or at least convince the community of molecular biologists that they were worth-while. Nebbishy, his hair brushed over his bald pate, he lived on the telephone and hopscotched the conference circuit, searching for new ideas and new talent.

In his office, Weinberg attempted to convince a graduate student called Mitch Goldfarb to carry out the work. Goldfarb already had the skills, having recently learnt the technique by taking sections of DNA from viruses and placing them in human cells. But Goldfarb told Weinberg that the experiment wouldn't work. After all, as the function of viruses is to slip inside animals cells, their genes were likely to be constructed to do so; however, Weinberg's idea was to take genes from mammalian cells, which were probably constructed quite differently. Without Goldfarb's agreement, Weinberg was unable to proceed: like other researchers in the lab, Goldfarb had his own small stipend from a charitable or educational source, and could not be ordered around by the lab's head.

Another problem was that many scientists believed that cancer was caused by the absence, rather than the presence, of particular genes. In this theory, the genes involved in cancer were like mechanical regulators, governing the speed at which cells duplicate; only when these genes were destroyed or damaged did uncontrolled cell proliferation begin. If that was the case, Goldfarb argued, then the whole transfection idea was misguided, for there would be no such thing as a cancer gene that could ever be inserted into a new cell. 'I was reluctant to forge ahead,' Goldfarb remembered, 'and Bob was reluctant to push.' But in the end, Weinberg's dogged enthusiasm persuaded Goldfarb to give it a try.

From a colleague, Weinberg procured some cancerous mouse kidney cells, a family of cells that had already existed for years, nourished, oxygenated and kept at the right temperature, each one replicating about once every day. They had originated from a healthy family of cells that had been bathed in chemicals to turn them malignant, such that they now formed disordered clusters in Petri dishes. Goldfarb took the cells, spun them in a liquidiser to destroy their structure and used various chemicals to isolate the long strands of DNA. Then he used a series of enzymes to cut up the ribbons of DNA into more manageable lengths, some of which he assumed would be the length of a gene. Next he added a chemical called calcium phosphate, which, as other researchers had shown, crystallised around the sections of DNA, wrapping it up into parcels to be delivered into cells.

Finally he mixed these DNA packages with millions of healthy mouse skin-like cells. The hope was that a DNA package from a cancerous cell would slip through a healthy cell's wall and splice itself into the functioning DNA. There was a certain crudeness to the technique; from previous experiments with viruses, Goldfarb knew that only once in every million cells was a single cancerous gene successfully transferred to a healthy cell – but as that was about the same as the contents of a couple of Petri dishes, he prepared more than twenty dishes to be certain of a result. After two weeks of incubation, Goldfarb studied the Petri dishes, but he saw no cancerous cell clusters. For weeks, he repeated the experiment, but nothing happened. So dismal was the progress that he would avoid Weinberg, for fear of having to talk about his failure. Other researchers in the lab looked on, convinced that the whole endeavour only demonstrated 'what kind of crazy lab Bob was running'.

After twenty-five attempts, however, miraculously clusters of cancerous cells appeared. There was only *one* successful result, so Goldfarb thought perhaps there had been some sort of mistake, or that a virus had accidentally contaminated the experiment. Yet even as Weinberg was contemplating what to do with this first tentative result, everyone in the field became convinced that transfection was a fraud.

In April 1978, Bob Weinberg went to a talk by Demetrios Spandidos, a young post-doctoral researcher from the University of Toronto. His compelling paper presented exactly the same conclusions that Weinberg had believed to be his own, though Spandidos had much more evidence. An article had already been accepted by the prestigious journal *Cell*, and so brilliant did the work appear to be that MIT was rumoured to be offering Spandidos a job. 'My depression deepened,' said Weinberg. 'My own research department was clearly intent on recruiting someone to do experiments very similar to those I had recently begun but not yet brought to fruition. It was a clear signal – a sharp slap in the face.'

But a few weeks after the talk, Spandidos's boss, Louis Siminovitch, accused Spandidos of inventing his results. Siminovitch simply did not believe that so many experiments could have been carried out in such a short time. Spandidos was asked to leave the laboratory and the paper was withdrawn from *Cell*. Although Spandidos vehemently denied any wrongdoing, and no independent audit was ever carried out, the whole scandal provoked feverish gossip among the close-knit community of molecular biology. As word spread, the idea of transfection, of inserting cellular genes into other cells, was also tarnished. Weinberg's results, which were already a little questionable, would now be viewed with even more scepticism.

Despite this, Weinberg was determined to press ahead. Mitch Goldfarb, though, had had enough. The single result after twenty-five attempts was not sufficiently compelling to continue on a project which he thought, in any case, would lead nowhere. So Weinberg was left to search for a new researcher to rise to this seemingly impossible challenge.

$\approx$

Taking a breather from visiting Dad, and flicking through family albums in the attic room of my parents' house, I came across photographs of Anita, the youngest of Mum's Danish cousins. In the pictures, she was about 25 years old, visiting us on holiday in the early 1970s. One depicted her sitting under a tree, the sunlight dappling the ground and cutting across her long brown hair. She was beautiful and looked as if she would live for ever.

The next album is of our family holiday to Denmark the following year. There are pictures of all Mum's other cousins, and their children. But Anita is absent: in those intervening months she had died of leukaemia. She was another member of the family, someone else with whom I shared some genes, to be added to the list.

Returning to the previous year's album, I gazed at her face. I realised that her death when I was only six had given me my first sense of cancer. Although my grandparents had died a few years earlier, I had been too young to understand. But during that holiday to Denmark, I remember catching, in fleeting scraps of conversation through doors that stood ajar, an empty hollow grief that would be forever associated with the disease.

&

With only a single tentative result, and without a researcher, Weinberg was forced to find someone else to continue trans-fecting mouse cancer genes into mouse cells. In the autumn of 1978, he was approached by a postgraduate student called Chiaho Shih, who was then assigned to another labora-tory in MIT. Shih's relationship with his current supervisor had soured, and, having come to Boston from Taiwan the year before, he now needed another laboratory in which to complete his doctorate. Yet although Shih was both morose and argumentative, he was more malleable than some of the lab's other researchers. 'When Shih arrived at the labora-tory,' thought Weinberg, 'he was at my mercy.' Though Shih tried to wriggle away from the deserted transfection project, Weinberg insisted it was the quid pro quo for working with him. So Shih began Weinberg's hare-brained scheme.

Throughout the autumn of 1978, although he followed exactly Goldfarb's method, he could not replicate the results. Again and again, he repeated the procedure, each time with slightly different conditions. After months of futility, he asked Weinberg to be assigned another project. Weinberg insisted he carry on for just a little longer. He suggested that they procure another set of healthy mouse cells, in case the originals had lost some of their life in the laboratory.

Just as Shih was about to despair, groups of cancerous cells began to appear on the Petri dishes. To persuade himself and Weinberg that it was not a fluke, Shih repeated the experi-ments, with different types of cells, and with various checks and balances to ensure that they were not seeing what they so dearly wanted to believe. As the evidence mounted, they realised that they were seeing the truth. Nothing as thrilling had ever happened to Weinberg in science. So, in June 1979, he reported his extraordinary findings at a conference in New Hampshire. 'My talk evoked no gasps from the audience, no exclamations of appreciation, no signs of enthusiasm,' remembered Weinberg. For although he believed in his data, his colleagues had the memories of fraud allegations fresh in their minds; they supposed that the cancerous clusters had been triggered by a contaminating virus, or that Shih had imagined that clusters of normal cells were really cancer. One scientist who attended Weinberg's talk scribbled, 'not very convincing demonstration' on his notes. 'It was all very anti-climactic,' Weinberg recollected. In any case, these had been mouse cancers, which might not have much relevance to human cancers.

Despite the lukewarm response, Weinberg continued to believe that he had discovered a method of profound importance, one that could be used to determine the function of certain genes, and that would, ultimately, be used on human cells. To reach that goal, he first decided to get Shih to try transfecting a cancer gene of a rat. Shih showed that these too could slip into healthy mouse cells; 'that was a turning point for me,' remembered Shih. For after one species barrier had been crossed, Shih thought, in due course he would be able to insert human genes into healthy mouse cells. When Weinberg took these new results to conferences, however, they too were dismissed. 'People made fun of Bob,' remembered one researcher. Next Weinberg instructed Shih to take the genes from a human cancer cell and insert them into an animal cell by the same transfection method.

In the spring of 1980, Shih borrowed some human cancer cells from a friend at the Dana-Farber Institute, in Boston, which were labelled as having been drawn from a man with bladder cancer years before. Back at the lab, Shih broke these cells apart in a liquidiser and filtered off the solid debris. Then he isolated the strands of DNA and mixed them with calcium phosphate to make the DNA packages for transfection. Finally, he mixed these DNA parcels with millions of healthy mouse cells. Two weeks later, when he looked down the microscope, he saw clusters of big, black cancer cells. Shih and Weinberg submitted a paper describing their success to *Nature*, on 22 September 1980, which unequivocally asserted that their experiment was 'the demonstration of these transmissible genes', the first direct evidence that a discrete section of human DNA could trigger cancer.

Yet the wider scientific community still regarded the technique of transfection with uncertainty, and they reserved judgement. The trouble was that while everybody could understand that Shih and Weinberg had snipped apart human DNA at the beginning of the process and then produced cancerous results at the end, the actual events that had taken place in the Petri dishes had been neither observed nor explained. For the sceptics, it was as if the pieces of a shredded plant had been flung on a patch of earth, and now it was unclear whether the resulting new plants had arisen from a single seed, parts of the stem or something that had been in the soil all along. Many of Weinberg's peers did not, therefore, endorse his conviction that his latest results would lead to the next step: the identification of a human cancer gene.

᠀

Forty-six weeks after diagnosis. With Dad declining, the thought that we might all be cursed by cancer became more intense. Exhausted from constant hospital visits, the ends of our nerves sanded down by the pushing and pulling of hope and despair, we all became contaminated by this fear. Even Mum, who had met cancer with the blasé confidence of a doctor who'd read all the journals, seemed to worry. And in the absence of a firm diagnosis of the primary site of the cancer, we found ourselves wondering if, like his parents, Dad had a pernicious form of colon cancer.

Searching through the family history, I found other

cancers. Of course Mum had had her breast cancer, but also her mother, Gerda, had undergone a radical mastectomy, a year after I was born, which was successful albeit at the cost of an arm that swelled up. As a child I remember staring at my grandmother's arms and wondering why one was encircled by so much flesh. Gerda's brother Bernard – my mother's favourite uncle – had also died from cancer of the lung, a few years before my sister's birth, and her name, Benita, supposedly alluded to his. He was remembered by the family as a sparkling raconteur who brought rooms to life. Of course there was Anita too, who had died of leukaemia in the 1970s. And on my father's side, not only my grandparents, but also my father's uncle, Robert, had died from the disease.

At the same time as we enumerated these various deaths, more and more relations passed in front of Dad's bed, cousins and in-laws coming to wish him well. It was as if he were holding a family party for both the living and the dead.

֍

At the beginning of 1980, having successfully sparked cancerous cell colonies after taking human DNA, packaging it up and transfecting it into cells, Weinberg still felt frustrated. For although he believed that one of the human genes had sparked the cancer, many others doubted him. 'I was tired of having to speak in a tentative voice, using the mealy-mouthed academic circumlocutions,' remembered Weinberg. At the same time, he did not really have the evidence to state his claim categorically. 'We trembled at the prospect of stating anything with total certainty, fearful that years down the road some enterprising graduate would find a flaw in what we said and then, god forbid, reveal us to be fools.'

The trouble was that transfection was such a crude technique. All that had been demonstrated was that one among many thousands of human cancer cell genes triggered cancer, but not which one or by what mechanism. The only way to overcome others' reluctance to accept what Weinberg now saw so clearly, was to identify the gene that caused cancer. As genes were too small to pull out and handle, this meant that to isolate the gene it had to be copied millions of times using the fairly new technique of cloning. 'We needed to move in close to these genes, so that we could finger them, feel their contours, know what they were really made of.'

While many sceptics doubted Weinberg's conclusions, a few appreciative researchers did believe him. They realised, like explorers grateful for new maps, that the method that he had pioneered was a sufficient foundation for the next step. So Michael Wigler at the Cold Springs Harbor Laboratory on Long Island had recruited Mitch Goldfarb, who had done some of the initial transfection work with Weinberg. For a while Bob Weinberg was upset that all the techniques he had developed were being transferred elsewhere: this was scientific betrayal. At the National Institutes of Health, a researcher called Mariano Barbacid also turned his lab's resources to cloning the human cancer gene; unlike the others, however, he did not have the heart to announce his intention: 'They were laughing at Bob, and I thought they would laugh at me too.'

'We were driven to this race,' remembers Weinberg. 'Not because we wanted to humiliate or beat other people but because I knew that people who did things second or third were dismissed as derivative or unoriginal.' Shih was given the task of cloning the human cancer gene, using tools that had rapidly improved in the five years since Weinberg had been chasing transfection. There were a series of enzymes, for instance, which could slice up the long filaments of DNA, cutting at particular points in the underlying protein patterns, like a child with a pair of scissors snipping at the threads of a ribbon. The shorter sections of DNA were not, however, always the length of a single gene. Too much enzyme and the DNA would be shredded into uselessness, too little and it would be left in pointlessly large parts. So for months, Shih failed to isolate or detect the gene. 'I was depressed the whole time,' remembers Shih. 'It was too hard. I thought it was stupid.'

At the same time, Weinberg heard that a researcher from Wigler's laboratory promised that the race was already won, and that a paper was about to be published in a scientific journal. On Long Island, they were using slightly different methods from Shih's. They had worked out how to use the enzymes to precisely slice the DNA, and had separated the section that triggered cancer from all the others. 'It was incredibly exciting. The feeling was like a mountaineer who reaches the summit,' remembers Wigler, 'and for the first time sees a new landscape.'

In the early autumn of 1981, Wigler and Goldfarb successfully cloned the human cancer gene. Shih managed to clone the gene also, a month or so later, though even years after the event Shih refused to believe that he had lost. 'We were beaten to the finish line by a nose,' wrote Weinberg later. 'Shih seemed to care, but no one else did.' Mariano Barbacid also produced the same result almost simultaneously. All three groups published their reports within days of each other in the spring of the following year. For the first time in history, researchers had identified and cloned a gene that was the essential mechanism of a human cancer, albeit only in laboratory cells. Shih and Weinberg wrote at the end of their paper, 'we have provided direct proof that the transforming sequences of a human carcinoma cell line are contained in a discrete contiguous segment of DNA'. After years of circumstantial evidence and tentative hypotheses, this was unequivocal concrete evidence.

❧

After two weeks of Dad lying in hospital, I couldn't seem to drive away the thought that his cancer was inherited. I looked at my sister and her children and wondered.

But Dad cautioned me against thinking that there was some kind of pattern, because although cancer was threaded through the generations of the family, there was little to imply that all of these separate diseases were connected. As he pointed out, one in three people will develop the disease in their lifetime, and one in four will die from it. With so many people afflicted, he said, it was hardly surprising that the scars ran through a group as large as our extended family.

§

'The excitement surrounding these human tumor genes will be short-lived since the isolations raise more questions than they answer,' wrote Weinberg shortly after the discovery that had shown that one particular gene could trigger cancer in a Petri dish. Like archaeologists who had just dug out an ancient artefact but knew nothing about it, they had no inkling as to how the gene worked or in what context it came alive. The mechanism by which the gene caused the disease still remained to be discovered.

Weinberg and his colleagues therefore retraced their steps to a landmark paper that had been published six years previously – and would eventually earn the authors, Michael Bishop and Harold Varmus, a Nobel Prize. This research had come to the conclusion that a gene from a virus that caused cancer in chickens apparently existed in all healthy birds, in some fishes and even humans. At the time, the discovery had seemed incredible, even shocking, for how could a healthy chicken have the cancer gene, scientists asked, without developing a tumour? Scientists had been wedded to the idea that viruses caused animal cancers by inserting a bad gene into healthy cells; Bishop and Varmus suggested, however, that cancers were caused when pre-existing genes were activated by something such as a virus, a chemical or radiation. This radically new idea supposed that the cancer gene existed in two subtly different formations, which laboratory tools could not distinguish between: one that was harmless and one that was cancerous. In healthy cells, they surmised, the potentially malignant gene played a central role in the life cycle of the cells; when it became damaged – accidentally, or by a chemical or radiation, for instance – the cell was transformed and uncontrollable growth resulted.

With the gene cloned, Weinberg began the search for the differences between the healthy and the harmless gene. He knew that the human bladder-cancer gene, like all genes, was a chain of so-called nucleic acid bases – adenines (As), guanines (Gs), cytosines (Cs) and thymines (Ts), the basic building blocks of life. And he had worked out that the bladder-cancer gene was 6,500 bases in length. Yet he did not know the exact sequence of the bases in either the good or the bad versions.

To find the difference, Weinberg assigned Cliff Tabin, an effervescent, confident postdoctoral researcher, to the task, Chiaho Shih having left the lab after receiving his doctorate. Tabin's first action was to take a stand against Weinberg's prejudices. Weinberg believed, along with most other scientists, that the problem of cancer was one of degree; that bad cells produced too much of an otherwise useful protein, as if a tap had been left on so that the cell spewed out an endless stream of what, under normal circumstances, would have been good. Weinberg held, therefore, that the error occurred in the part of the gene that regulated how much protein was produced. At group meetings, Weinberg would excitedly explain how they were going to find the mutation in this specific part of the gene. But Tabin profoundly disagreed. Cancer, for him, was about the creation of an entirely new mechanism. The mutation created a new protein that instructed the cell to divide, and divide again, as if a switch had been flicked rather than a dial turned.

Although Weinberg thought he already knew the answer, Cliff Tabin – and various other people in the lab – proved him wrong, showing that a new protein was indeed created.

This insight would have profound consequences for medical researchers, as, in years to come, it would be much easier to block a single protein than to regulate the level of one that already exists and already has a useful function. This insight is fundamental to the current boom in research for drugs against cancer genes.

If the gene was producing a new kind of protein, there remained a question: what was the aberration in the gene that produced the bad protein? Weinberg reckoned the difference between the good gene and the bad gene would be a significant number of the 6,500 nucleic acid bases, because a complicated disease such as cancer would require large amounts of information, hundreds of bases, rather than just one or two. So, Cliff Tabin began to narrow down the area where the error had occurred, first to a thousand nucleic acid bases, then to a length 350 bases long. As they were homing in on the error, Weinberg knew that Michael Wigler and Mariano Barbacid were also attempting to discover the extent of the mutation. 'I was getting desperate,' remembered Weinberg. 'Having come that far, the final step was about to elude us.'

Hoping to accelerate the research, Weinberg began looking for talent and expertise from outside his laboratory. At a conference, he met Ravi Dhar from the National Institutes of Health in Bethesda, Maryland, who had developed a new technique using X-rays that could number and name the patterns of nucleic bases in any gene. Weinberg persuaded Dhar to work on his project, by agreeing that Dhar's name would appear on any eventual scientific paper. Dhar took the lengths of 350 nucleic bases from both the good and the bad genes back to his laboratory. In the summer of 1982, Dhar flew to Boston with the first results. He had discovered that the mutation was the smallest difference between two genes, an alteration in just a single nucleic base. Once again, Weinberg refused to believe it. It seemed so fantastical. So Dhar returned to Bethesda, where he re-analysed the error, and each time the aberration was the same. The mistake, the difference between the healthy and cancerous gene, was so small it was as if just one letter was out of place in a single-spaced text seven pages in length. At the same time, Mariano Barbacid also discovered this tiny blemish. Both papers were published in the journal *Nature* on 11 November 1982. 'It is one of the most startling discoveries so far in the long and frustrating search for an understanding of cancer,' proclaimed the journal's normally austere editorial.

For almost two centuries, scientists had been investigating the human body with greater and greater magnification, but no one had ever imagined that the journey would end up so precisely at the gates of the disease. As *Nature*'s editorial put it, Weinberg's work was 'as nice an illustration as there could be of how logic can triumph over incredulity'. If the mutation that Weinberg and his colleagues had discovered caused cancer in the average human body with its 10 million million cells – each human having about 35,000 genes, and each gene comprising a chain of some thousands of nucleic acid bases – it was as if a single-letter typing mistake had occurred in just one copy of *Hamlet*, with the result that every work of Shakespeare in the entire world was destroyed. Not since Virchow's discovery of cancer's cellular pathology in 1855 had an event in cancer science seemed to be so funda-mental and revolutionary. What was perhaps remarkable, something many newspapers picked up on, was just how quickly the transformation had taken place. 'Human cancer research is now moving forward faster than anyone thought possible,' said Weinberg in the *New York Times*.

According to some historians of science, the cloning of the human gene and the discovery of the malignant mutation was a dramatic revolution in the history of cancer. Before, there had been much confusion about the mechanism of cancer and many competing theories, but after 1982 there was a new paradigm, which most scientists subscribed to. The change had occurred, according to these historians, because of a perfect match between a testable hypothesis – that genes were the motor of cancer – and a new set of tools, such as the enzymes to slice DNA and the methods to replicate a gene. Until then there had been much to suggest that such a theory was indeed correct; but only when it became possible to manipulate and clone genes could the idea be proved. That three independent teams arrived at the same conclusion almost simultaneously had occurred because each had adopted these new techniques before they were widely disseminated. Thereafter the scientific community began to adopt the new paradigm of the genetic forces of cancer.

꙾

Forty-six and a half weeks after diagnosis. Fifteen days after hospital readmission. I sat on the edge of Dad's bed. He was too tired to read, and as a result he did not have much to say for himself. So, I told him the story of the discovery of the genetic basis of cancer. Dad listened to my enthusiasm. He nodded when I told him that the genetic paradigm was the most important discovery in the history of cancer during the last century.

Yet he raised an objection. He said that he knew that it was fashionable to characterise science as a series of great revolutions in which fundamental theories were forged; and that in between these so-called paradigm shifts scientists incrementally embroider these grand theories. Dad pointed me to *The Structure of Scientific Revolutions* by Thomas Kuhn, which was on his bookshelf, in which this idea of the process of science had first been formulated. But, as a scientist, Dad did not think that was how science really worked. For him, the events of 1982 were just one point on a continuum that included such discoveries as the double-helix structure of DNA in 1953, as well as the various methods to manipulate genes and slice strands of DNA, and that stretched forward in time as more detail became known about the genetic basis of cancer.

Dad gently chided me for believing in the paradigm-shifting theory of scientific progress. He said that it had only become so popular because it happened to coincide with the demands of journalists and film-makers who wanted to make neat stories, in which rapid change occurred, from the slow and gradual process of science. In any case, he said, many historians doubted the argument put forward in *The Structure of Scientific Revolutions*. One only had to look at another of Thomas Kuhn's books, he said, about Copernicus, which described slow advances made by drawing on the work of many individuals, to understand truly how science worked.

❦

No matter how science is perceived to progress, 1982 was an *annus mirabilis* of cancer medicine. Having identified the mutation of the human bladder-cancer gene, Bob Weinberg also unified the disparate fields of cancer research when one of his researchers, Louis Parada, discovered that the human cancer gene was indeed the same as one from an animal cancer virus. 'My first reaction was one of disappointment,' remembered Weinberg, for he had thought that he had been forging an entirely new field, whereas, in fact, he had been studying a gene that had already long been identified. The same malfunction could also be created in some animal cells by bathing them in chemicals. As a consequence, Weinberg soon realised that this 'was one of those rare, fleeting moments in science when a connection is forged between two seemingly disconnected entities, each interesting in its own right'. Where once cancer was thought of as an incredibly complex disease, appearing in many different forms, caused differently by radiation, chemicals and viruses, there was now a much simpler explanation: there existed just a few genes whose malfunction, caused by any of these processes, could trigger the disease across many species. And all cancers had genetic faults at their heart.

In the following years, the papers by Weinberg, Barbacid and Wigler were cited by hundreds of others. Although they had identified the first human cancer gene, there were many others to discover. Very quickly, other research teams raced to find genes that triggered cancer in different locations, from the breast to the stomach. The list of genes that play some part in human cancer now has hundreds of entries.

In contradiction to the first discoveries, some of these genes trigger the disease by their presence, because they send, for instance, an insistent signal that the cell must divide. Others are dangerous through their absence: when they are present they spend their lives slowing down cell division, but when they are knocked out completely or subtly damaged, the changes that lead to the disease begin. Although in 1982 it appeared to some as if the mechanism of cancer could be simple insofar as it required the malfunction of just a single gene, in subsequent years the picture has become more complicated.

In fact, very few if any cancers are the result of only a singular error. The current orthodoxy is that most cancers arise when a single cell accumulates a series of errors during the course of its life. Chronic myeloid leukaemia appears to begin with just one mistake, for instance, but becomes fatal only when other errors are made. Colon polyps generally occur when a few genes mutate, and they turn into cancer when a few more are damaged. The requirement for a series of genes to mutate is why cancer is predominantly a disease of old age, for only after years, after the accumulated degradation of the genes of a single cell, will it become dangerous.

Yet the picture that has emerged is not only one of complexity. There are some genes, notably the one cloned by Weinberg, Wigler and Barbacid called *ras*, which contribute to the development of a range of cancers. Another called P53, for example, contributes to more than 50 per cent of all cancers. For the first time, the many different types of cancer appear to have some shared characteristics. And if the same cancerous gene is active in many different cancers, then the search for treatments ought not to be quite so daunting.

&.

After three weeks, Dad remained in hospital. For a moment there was stasis; he was immobile, periodically in pain, neither recovering nor declining. As a family we calmed down. We also grew a little optimistic, believing that he would soon be out of hospital, at home among his books.

We became more realistic about our genetic inheritance, too, although in truth we couldn't begin to know whether he had bequeathed bad genes, because we still didn't know where the primary tumour was; none of the imaging technologies available would reveal it. When we considered the most likely place – a tumour in the prostate – the risk of it having some inherited component was less than 10 per cent. Yet even if Dad had inherited the disease, there were likely to be other factors, such as the chemicals in smoke or in some vegetables, or such as radiation, that had contributed to the damage to his cells. Some of the damage would also have come about because of random accidents: when a cell copies its own genes very occasionally – like a tired photocopier, where the paper is crinkled or the toner running short – the replica is incomplete or a little damaged.

Dad's equanimity towards the bubbling breathing-apparatus of the patient in the next bed, or the other disturbances of the ward, was matched by a stoicism towards our common genes. For he believed that even if a particular genetic blemish had been passed to him from his father, there was no telling whether in another part of his body, at another stage of his life, it had served to protect his cells, or given his mind a particular characteristic that would not otherwise have been there. After years of not knowing his body, he seemed at last to be coming to terms with the idea that he was one being undivided, the good and bad consequences of the actions of 10 million million cells.

Prevention:

making your own luck

THREE AND A HALF WEEKS after arriving in hospital, Dad was becoming more incapable. When one day he needed some help to leave his bed for the toilet, I called a nurse. Because he was large and heavy, the nurse told me that she needed the help of a colleague, who was currently busy elsewhere. Half an hour later, I made the request again and soon two nurses came trotting down the ward. Dad sat up, and the nurses took his legs from underneath the bedclothes and moved them towards the edge of the bed, twisting his body. He winced from the pain, as his skin was so fragile that it grazed on bed sheets. Eventually, like a parachutist preparing for a jump, he was ready to descend, a nurse on either side of him. He put his feet down, steadying himself on their shoulders. But his knees could no longer support his weight. The nurses had been trained not to sacrifice their backs. So they gracelessly let him drop. Like a wounded soldier, he crumbled on to his knees and then on to the floor. Transfixed, I was unable to move, unsure of what I could do. He flailed around, failing to find any purchase on the shiny linoleum floor of the ward. A nurse closed the curtains around his bed, as his elasticised bedsocks kicked against the air. His powerlessness reinforced my gathering feeling of bleakness. After some minutes, a winch was brought and they hoisted him out of trouble.

That evening, I recounted Dad's fall to my sister, Benita, on the phone. It silenced us. For a moment we both listened to the dead electronic hiss, neither of us able to utter a word for fear that we would betray our feelings.

Thirty-one months older than me, Benita had always been on the other end of a phone whenever necessary, more stable and stronger than me. Yet in the swirling fear and sadness of Dad's decline I worried about her too – for Mum had had breast cancer, as had her mother, and sister.

Although breast cancer ran in the family, I learnt that my sister's risk was very small. Typing the details of her age, our family and when she had her children into a website that calculates the risk, I discovered that she had an 8 in 1,000 chance of developing the disease within the next five years. Even five years hence, her risk would only increase to 13 in 1,000.

These were tiny risks, but they were rising. And there was every possibility that they had some kind of familial character. Perhaps we carried the gene called BRCA1, which sits on the seventeenth chromosome in all the cells of the body, or perhaps we had another called BRCA2. The Ashkenazi Jewish heritage of my grandparents apparently increased the likelihood that we were carrying these mutations. It has been estimated that between 5 and 10 per cent of all breast cancers have one of these two malevolent factors involved, and that women who carry the gene have between a 35 to 80 per cent chance of developing the disease at some point in their lifetimes. There is also some evidence that BRCA2 plays an important role in the development of male prostate cancer.

Imagined or real, these were the Damoclean swords that hung above our family. Although Dad and I had spent so long talking about how to treat the disease, he also wondered if there was a way to avert it entirely.

The war on cancer's failure to reduce mortality rates had, by the mid 1980s, cast doubt on the strategy of rushing to discover new treatments. In consequence, policy makers on both sides of the Atlantic began to focus on prevention and the medical truism that this – in the form of clean water, vaccinations and tobacco control – had always saved more lives than clinical treatments. Screening programmes, such as for cervical cancer, had long existed, but there was now renewed enthusiasm for them: in 1987, for example, the National Cancer Institute recommended routine breast cancer screening for women in their forties; and in Britain, a National Breast Cancer Screening Programme was begun in 1988 for women aged 50–64.

At much the same time, there was the lure of chemoprevention – the idea that cancer might itself be prevented by giving drugs to healthy individuals, by increasing or reducing the amounts of certain chemicals, such as vitamins or hormones, in the body, so that the mechanisms that trigger cancer would be slowed.

Leading the charge, in America, was a professor at the University of Pittsburgh named Bernard Fisher. Then in his early seventies, Fisher was already a kind of hero for many in the field of cancer medicine because, after more than twenty years of campaigning, he had shown that the radical mastectomy, which included the removal of at least one chest muscle and some lymph nodes, was normally only necessary for the most extreme kinds of breast cancer. Although the procedure had been widely promoted by surgeons for almost a century, Fisher had demonstrated that it was unnecessarily invasive, and that a smaller operation called the lumpectomy was at least as successful. His research method was to track thousands of women after they had undergone one of these procedures in the years following their operations – results which he published in his landmark paper in the *New England Journal of Medicine* in 1985.

As a result, Fisher found himself a fellow traveller with the growing movement of women's activists who had long believed that surgeons had been overenthusiastically cutting into their bodies. At the same time, the medical profession embraced him when that year he received the prestigious Albert Lasker Memorial Prize.

Years later, Fisher would characterise this moment with a quotation from F. Scott Fitzgerald: 'Show me a hero and I'll write you a tragedy.'

Bernard Fisher's Breast Cancer Prevention Trial was launched in June 1992, with a flurry of publicity. It followed a smaller British trial that had already piqued the interest of cancer doctors. Other large trials were underway testing chemicals that ordinarily appeared in food, such as beta carotene, but Fisher's trial was a step into a new realm as he had chosen to give an existing drug called tamoxifen daily to enormous numbers of *healthy* women. As the study offered the hope of a new kind of medicine, the director of the US Government's National Cancer Institute, Samuel Broder, had declared it a priority, and had allocated $68 million over the following five years to the effort. Issuing press releases and taking out advertising, the 268 centres involved had soon recruited thousands of the 16,000 women required.

Tamoxifen had already proved itself as a drug for breast cancer treatment. By blocking the female hormone oestrogen from acting in cells, it stopped a signal for cell duplication being communicated, thus preventing lesions from becoming lumps, and lumps becoming tumours. Taken after breast cancer surgery, it reduced the risk of the disease recurring in the majority of patients by 50 per cent, according to British research authored by Michael Baum and Jack Cuzick and subsequently followed up by Bernard Fisher and other international researchers. At the time Fisher was contemplating using the drug for prevention, my mother and millions of other women were taking it daily in the years after their operations.

In fact, the idea of giving tamoxifen to healthy women had been triggered by results of the first British trials of the drug on women recovering from surgery. In these trials, a woman taking the drug had about a third likelihood of developing the disease in their healthy breast as was normal. Would the results be the same for healthy women?

Fisher believed that the 175,000 breast cancer cases diagnosed annually in America represented just the 'tip of the iceberg'. In addition there were many more women who had some kind of aberration in their breasts that had not yet been detected. And tamoxifen seemed to have the power, he thought, to stop these defective cells from duplicating. Fisher promised that the success of the trial would result in 'drastic, paradigmatic change in the treatment of breast cancer', from treating the well-developed disease, to catching and treating it even before cells took on the identity of tumours.

The trial became entangled in controversy even before it could begin. One of Fisher's principal opponents was the National Women's Health Network, a Washington consumer health lobby group that launched campaigns and nurtured legislators from cramped offices next to a fast-food restaurant. One of its directors, Adriane Fugh-Berman, had previously supported tamoxifen as a treatment, for in what she viewed as the 'slash-and-burn' world of cancer therapy, it was relatively benign with limited side effects ranging from hot flushes, vaginal discharge, irregular periods to skin rashes; the more serious risks of uterine and liver cancers were rare. 'The risk/benefit ratio for women with a life-threatening cancer,' she argued, 'definitely favours Tamoxifen.'

However, the Breast Cancer Prevention Trial was planning to give the drug not to ill patients but to healthy women. 'The acceptable risks for the sick are not acceptable risks for the well,' wrote Fugh-Berman, who saw no reason to 'medicalize' women who had reported no illnesses or to subject them to any 'known risks, for an unknown benefit'. She objected because the predictions for the trial meant that for every 1,000 healthy women, 983 would take the drug, potentially suffer side effects, but gain no benefit as the drug would probably only prevent the disease in less than half of those 17 women per 1,000 that would have developed it.

A drug-based strategy for prevention, according to Fugh-Berman, would therefore set a worrying historical precedent. Up to then, the twentieth century had seen only preventative measures, such as public health messages against smoking or in favour of exercise, which had been harmless; and when they had involved a degree of risk, such as vaccinations against polio, the benefits had been clear. A physician herself, Fugh-Berman believed that the idea of giving drugs to the healthy had been developed because those organising the trial were not tentative, risk-averse public health doctors but oncologists. 'They are on the frontier, they are extremely confident,' she said. 'But they are used to risky therapies.'

At the heart of this controversy was a conflict between two of the central principles of medical ethics. On the one hand, there was the principle of beneficence, as asserted by doctors in their Hippocratic Oath: 'I will prescribe regimens for the good of my patients.' On the other, was the Hippocratic injunction that a doctor should 'never do any harm'. Yet doctors had long understood that the risk of harm was a central part of medical practice, and could be balanced by benefit. The small dangers of infection and bleeding from surgery, for instance, were usually outweighed by its success in treating patients. For the advocates of the Breast Cancer Prevention Trial, therefore, tamoxifen's ability to save lives more than balanced the probable risk of side effects and fatalities. By contrast, the trial's opponents emphasised the categorical imperative of doing no harm.

One of the first women to be recruited was Renee Rauch, who was based in Howell Township, in New Jersey. Then aged 47, she had watched her mother die after undergoing two radical mastectomies. 'It was a terrible, frightening thing to witness,' she remembered. 'After all her pain and suffering, she was dead at sixty-eight. I knew that if there was any chance to avoid my mother's experience with breast cancer, I'd take a shot at it.' Through her work as a hospital clerk, she heard that the trial was beginning at a nearby hospital and went to an induction. There she was told about some of the risks and benefits. 'I think nothing would have dissuaded me from taking part. I believe that it's important to participate in clinical trials. And I thought it might really help.' With her own two daughters then in their twenties, Rauch also hoped that the research might prove useful to them.

To be accepted on the trial, Renee Rauch had to show that she had a slightly elevated level of risk of developing cancer. So she was asked about her age, the date of her first period, if she had children and, if so, when she had given birth, whether her mother or sister had the disease, and if she had ever had any biopsies for invasive cancer. Putting these variables into existing models of risk, Rauch's was calculated to be above the trial's threshold.

Rauch began taking the drug in September 1992. Although the trial was supposed to be blind – in that half of the women were to be given the drug and the others a sugar-pill placebo – Renee Rauch immediately realised that she had been given tamoxifen. 'Since I've been on the program I've been getting hot flushes that wake me twice a night without fail. My periods have become irregular. But I'm very determined to do this because my fear was so great,' she told a reporter.

So convinced was Rauch by the possibilities that she tried to persuade her sister, Evie Pritzker, who lived in Illinois, to begin the trial also. Pritzker was more at risk of developing cancer, as she had once had a biopsy and was three years older than Rauch; however, Pritzker felt very differently about the trial. 'She was scared off by the possible side effects,' said Rauch at the time. Pritzker also felt that to take tamoxifen when she did not need it would prevent her from taking it as a treatment should she ever develop breast cancer in the future. Over the telephone, Rauch remonstrated with her older sister. But to little avail.

The sisters were able to make their own choices. Yet many participants were not able to make clearly informed decisions, as the doctors administering the trial in clinics around the country had, in general, underestimated risks, according to an investigation by a congressman named Donald Payne. Entitled 'Are Healthy Women Put At Risk By Federally Funded Research?', the hearing was held by his committee in October 1992. 'After attending a meeting at our local hospital ... I was concerned about the paucity of the information provided,' complained one prospective participant, Susan Blake Rowland, of Hillsborough, California. 'We were given very little literature and the possible side effects were discussed only generally.'

The most startling discovery of the enquiry was that more than two-thirds of the institutions taking part in the study had watered down at least one of the key points of the model consent form drawn up by Fisher, the National Cancer Institute and the manufacturer of tamoxifen, Zeneca. About half of them, for instance, had minimized the risk of liver cancer; and almost a quarter had changed 'three predicted deaths' caused by blood clots among the 16,000 participants in the trial to 'three predicted cases'. As a consequence, the administrators of the National Institutes of Health resolved to tighten up and audit consent forms more thoroughly in the future.

Journalists also failed to outline clearly the subtle calculi of risk and benefit. It was as if they were more used to reporting cancer medicine using old formulae: either the latest scientific breakthrough was breathlessly sold as a new cure, or an industrial hazard or a household consumable was claimed as a new danger. These tropes had been changing: the long-running debate about the best method of breast cancer surgery – mastectomy or lumpectomy – had been widely covered, many magazines and newspapers carrying stories, and angry first-person narratives, demanding that women ought to be given the correct information and then be allowed to choose which procedure was practised on their own bodies. At the same time, some of the archaic taboos were being challenged. The *New York Times Magazine*, for instance, placed the image of a woman after a mastectomy on its cover in the autumn of 1993. But when it came to the dilemmas that were now being posed by tamoxifen and in other areas of modern cancer medicine, the complexity was often lost in the search for a good headline. Men like Bernard Fisher despaired: 'I still do not appreciate the virtue of public debate via sound bites in the media,' Fisher wrote around this time, 'because this inappropriately shapes the public opinion.'

Even as the trial was progressing, the balance of risk was changing as new information became available. In the autumn of 1993, there was an unexpected result from an entirely different but nonetheless relevant trial, which was also being run by Bernard Fisher. In this trial, 2,639 women had been taking tamoxifen after breast cancer surgery treatment to prevent recurrence. Of those, twenty-three had contracted uterine cancer, and four had died of it.

These results meant that six out of every thousand women who were taking part in the Breast Cancer Prevention Trial would be likely to develop uterine cancer within five years, although few of those would die as the disease was relatively easy to treat by the removal of the uterus. Fisher had originally advised prospective patients that taking tamoxifen would not result in 'deaths from uterine cancers'; however, he now changed the consent form to read 'uterine cancer can be a life-threatening disease'.

Some of Fisher's colleagues believed the scales had been tipped, with the risks of participation now outweighing the benefits for women who had little likelihood of developing breast cancer. As a result, doctors at the University of Kansas began to discourage women who had a very low risk of developing breast cancer from taking part in the trial – 'though we certainly wouldn't refuse them,' said one. However, Fisher maintained that 'We have conducted a risk-benefit analysis, and we still find that there is a benefit going ahead with the trial.' Other than a small article in the trade journal *Science*, the recalculation of risk slipped quietly beneath the media radar and was even missed by the National Women's Health Network. Had not Bernard Fisher been propelled into the national spotlight, the Breast Cancer Prevention Trial would have continued.

In the fourth week of hospital, Dad reminded me of a time when I was quite young. We were on holiday somewhere, and we had been playing games of chance. The first game involved two dice; the winner was the one who more often guessed the sum of the two faces before the dice were rolled. Dad's big hand rolled the dice, and again and again he won, because he knew the odds. As we continued to play and I began to master the game, he changed the rules. He added a die. Then another. I became more and more frustrated, and so Dad began to teach me the simple rules of probability: that seven is the most likely score of two dice thrown together, that a coin tossed after many throws is equally likely to fall heads or tails. And then he began to let me win.

He taught me a lesson that day: it is bad to make single bets. There are good odds that fifty out of a hundred coin tosses will come up heads, but you have to rely on luck if you bet on a single toss of the coin.

Thirty years later, he reminded me about the games because he thought they had a parallel in the prevention of cancer. Any preventative strategy relies upon reducing the odds of individuals developing the disease across the whole population

– the equivalent of many tosses of the coin; but individuals can only take preventative bets on themselves, on just one event, so they are faced with difficult decisions. If they adopt preventative strategies, such as taking tamoxifen, in order to lessen their odds of developing cancer, they are also relying on luck. For every 1,000 taking tamoxifen, 984 would see no benefit, 8 would develop cancer, and only another lucky 8 would see their cancer prevented, on the basis of the predicted results of the trial.

❧

On Sunday 13 March 1994, the *Chicago Tribune* ran a front-page story with the headline 'FRAUD IN BREAST CANCER STUDY', the central allegation of which was that a doctor named Roger Poisson based in Montreal had 'falsified and fabricated' the medical records of ninety-nine patients he had enrolled in Bernard Fisher's breast cancer surgery trials – including the trial that had shown the lumpectomy was usually preferable to radical mastectomy. Written by an acclaimed investigative reporter named John Crewdson, the story alleged that Poisson had been so enthusiastic about signing women up to the trials that he had lied about their case histories.

The *Tribune* article led to a cascade of further stories in the *New York Times,* the *Chicago Sun Times,* the *San Francisco Chronicle* and virtually every other American newspaper. In the following weeks, the furore blossomed. Each day brought slight iterations to the original allegations. And within a month the scandal was being reported as if it were the biggest in medical history.

These stories were, at first, not about Fisher's Breast Cancer Prevention Trial. Rather Crewdson's most damaging revelation was that 16 per cent of the case histories that formed the basis of Fisher's landmark 1985 *New England Journal of Medicine* paper about breast cancer surgery had been contributed by Poisson, although not all of them were inaccurate.

But consequently, Crewdson said, 'the precise effect of the Montreal fraud on these and related studies remains unclear', the implication being that it was still not known whether a lumpectomy or a radical mastectomy was indeed the better surgical strategy for a woman suffering from breast cancer.

In the previous year, the US Government's Office of Research Integrity had investigated the fraud when it had been brought to light by the checks and balances of the drug trial. But it had issued no report, nor widely publicised that there was little to worry about, nor had Fisher published a re-analysis of the results. With the fraud now public, though, a spokesman for the Office of Research Integrity said, 'We are concerned that we might have a public health crisis.'

In fact, most scientists quickly realised that the fraud had accounted for an irrelevantly small number of patients; and there were reports of other trials in Scandinavia, Britain and Japan that confirmed Fisher's findings about the greater benefit of lumpectomies, so that his report was not the sole basis on which patients and their doctors were making decisions between a lumpectomy and radical mastectomy.

Yet the media continued to stoke the scandal, and the focus shifted to Bernard Fisher himself. For although it was the Canadian doctor, Poisson, who had invented the crucial medical details, Fisher and the US Government's Office of Research Integrity had damned themselves in the eyes of the media when they failed to announce the fraud or their subsequent investigation of it. And Fisher was furthermore accused of failing to deliver a corrected version of the original paper with a re-analysis of the numbers so that the fraud could be cleaned from the results. 'If breast cancer patients are now fearful and sceptical,' a *New York Times* editorial stated, 'the researchers have only themselves to blame.'

One of the causes of this distrust had been a series of scientific misconduct cases brought to centre stage by a congressman named John Dingell, who now joined the fray with the promise to hold a congressional hearing about breast cancer fraud. He said, 'this episode is yet another example of how scientific misconduct coupled with inadequate Federal Government response can undermine efforts to improve health and safety of the public'.

Fisher's voice went unheard in the ferocious media assault. 'It interfered with every aspect of my life. That was so tragic,' remembers Fisher. 'It was a waste of energy and time.'

Three weeks after the original publication of the *Chicago Tribune* report, Fisher was drowning in recriminations. And those funding the Breast Cancer Prevention Trial at the National Cancer Institute began to distance themselves from him. Claiming that he had failed to submit data to them for auditing, they sent him a sharply worded letter demanding that the data about breast cancer surgery be re-analysed. And at much the same time, Cindy Pearson of the National Women's Health Network seized the opportunity to re-open questions about the legitimacy of giving tamoxifen to healthy women. Other critics also joined in. Slowly the focus of the media storm shifted from the efficacy of the lumpectomy to reports on the numbers of patients who had developed uterine cancers after taking tamoxifen, results that Fisher had discovered some months before.

Fisher responded with the words, 'These criticisms have been going on since day one when the Tamoxifen trial started. [But] if the trial were to stop this would be a great tragedy for the women in the trial.' The director of the National Cancer Institute, Samuel Broder, was amazed at the ferocity of the assault, as the women's health activists, the hungry press and contrarian scientists collided with unprecedented force. Fearing that public support would ebb away, and that women would stop taking tamoxifen, Broder asked the University of Pittsburgh to replace Fisher as the head of the Breast Cancer Prevention trial. 'We did that to make sure that the trial could proceed with the assurance to the public,' remembers Broder. 'The study was transcendently important to me. And one cannot proceed in a democracy without the endorsement of the public.' At the same time, patient recruitment was suspended pending a full investigation.

The frenzy surrounding Fisher reached its peak on 13 April 1994 when John Dingell convened his Committee of Oversight in Congress. The star witness – whose face adorned the front page of the next day's *New York Times* – was a political lobbyist named Jill Lea Sigal who had met Dingell at a fund-raising dinner and had been given the opportunity to testify about her own experience of being a breast cancer patient: 'My anger and outrage that a doctor [Poisson] could possibly engage in such gross scientific fraud was surpassed only by my disbelief when I learned that the National Cancer Institute, an instrument of the US government, knew about the falsified data three years ago and deliberately did not give it widespread publicity.' The question she asked was 'How many women during these three years made a decision about their surgery, as I did, based on this study?'

The committee's witnesses also criticised the Breast Cancer Prevention Trial itself: Cindy Pearson, of the National Women's Health Network, said that it was 'originally a bad idea [that] is well on the way to becoming a disaster'. The drug tamoxifen, she said, might be good medicine for women with breast cancer, but 'to healthy women it is closer to poison'. As if the bile of the general media was not enough for Bernard Fisher to contend with, over the following days, critical editorials appeared in both the *New England Journal of Medicine* and the *Journal of the American Medical Association*.

§♣

After seeing Dad almost immobile in a hospital bed, I went in search of his old spirit in his workshop. When I entered the garage, there remained the smell of old ink and turpentine. The fluorescent light flickered on above the Victorian printing machines. One still had shiny black ink cloaking its rollers, as if the diligent craftsman in charge had just slipped out for dinner.

Dad's places always seemed to be in a kind of chaos: papers, trays of lead type, half-read magazines, ink and piles of beautiful papers delicately balanced into towers. He claimed to know the exact location of anything one might request. There had always been a patina of dust sprinkled across the objects, but now the press and the papers were wrapped in carpets of fibrous grime. In a paper cabinet, rather than beautiful watermarked leaves, I found only a tangled mess of shredded paper, where a mouse had made a home. Everywhere the absence of Dad's energy had allowed his creative disorganisation to slip into a dirty mess. For as much as chaos was taking over his body, so disarray was also enveloping the things he loved.

I opened a drawer of type. Once Dad's big hands had placed each tiny lead letter in the correct order, and the letters had become words, and he had placed the lines together to make pages ready for printing. Now the orderly lines of letters had fallen sideways, and the words were in a jumble. In other drawers, the muddle repeated itself as thousands of letters fell over themselves. There were still some lines of poetry and aphorisms, and even some pages of sentences, but there was also much nonsense. It made me think of the errors in the patterns of nucleic acids that now formed some of his genes.

꧁

The controversy surrounding the Breast Cancer Prevention Trial was mirrored in other debates about cancer prevention, such as the efficacy of routine mammography screening. In January 1997, the US National Cancer Institute convened a meeting of twelve impartial experts with the aim of arriving at a consensus on whether women under the age of 50 should have routine mammograms. The group spent weeks reading hundreds of research reports in preparation, then called thirty speakers to discuss the data during their three-day meeting. There was plenty of evidence to pick through, as almost half a million women had taken part in trials to determine the benefits of screening programmes during the previous thirty years.

The conclusion of the panel was that 'the data currently available do not warrant a universal recommendation for mammography for all women in their forties'. The argument was supported by evidence from thousands of women which demonstrated that breast cancer screening saved the lives of women in their fifties but appeared to have little if any effect for women in their forties. At best, the panel estimated that as little as one life might be extended for every 2,500 women in their forties screened for a decade.

They also pointed out the small dangers linked to screening. About a third of all women would, at some point in their forties, be told that they had something that looked like cancer, only for a biopsy to prove that it was not cancer. These so-called 'false positives', caused by the crudeness of the technology, would, the panel thought, bring unnecessary anxiety and fear to large numbers of women. Similarly, some women would have to face the risks of medical intervention with little benefit, because mammography would identify abnormalities that would appear to be precursors to cancer but that would never develop to be invasive or life-threatening. Finally, there was a small chance – one which the panel estimated to be less than 1 in 10,000 – that the radiation from mammography would induce breast cancer rather than prevent it.

Because this equation of risk and benefit was so finely drawn, the panel recommended that 'Each woman should decide for herself whether to undergo mammography. Her decision may be based not only on an objective analysis of the scientific evidence and consideration of her individual medical history, but also on how she perceives and weighs each potential risk and benefit, the values she places on each, and how she deals with uncertainty.' By giving responsibility to the women themselves, the panel had effectively elevated the ethical principle of autonomy – the right to choose one's own treatment – above any other. In a world that was increasingly opposed to doctors paternalistically telling patients what they ought to do, such a strategy should have won them many friends.

Yet the recommendation surprised many. Richard Klausner, the director of the National Cancer Institute, said at a press conference that he was 'shocked' by the decision, in particular because the panel had omitted to emphasise that screening reduced mortality. Similarly, a radiologist publicly stated that withholding screening was 'tantamount to a death sentence', adding, 'I grieve for them.' One Harvard doctor called the panel's decision 'fraudulent', even though the report had meticulously set out such evidence as there was. The media reported the event with typically exaggerated prose: the *Chicago Tribune* ran an article with the headline 'NEW MAMMOGRAM REPORT LEAVES WOMEN ADRIFT'. On 4 February 1997, the US Senate unanimously passed a resolution that urged the National Cancer Institute to recommend mammograms for women in their forties. With mounting pressure, the National Cancer Institute convened another committee and, on 27 March 1997, issued a statement that women in their forties should indeed be screened every one to two years.

Even though there had been no new evidence, the slight beneficence of mammograms was now promoted above the principle of patient autonomy. There was some irony that some twenty years earlier the women's health movement had vigorously campaigned against doctors who took decisions on their patients' behalf. Now a disappointed editorial in the *New England Journal of Medicine* proclaimed that women ought to be allowed to make their own decisions based on their 'private and personal feelings about health outcomes and not on the loudest or most prestigious voice'.

ᛒ

A month after Bernard Fisher resigned, in 1994, the storm abated, allowing him to begin slowly rebuilding his reputation. He appeared at a second hearing of the Dingell committee a few months after the first, where he accepted his share of the responsibility for the administrative deficiencies that occurred, and convincingly rebutted the allegation that he had withheld the information from the women. 'Perhaps,' he said, 'my passionate attention to the science overshadowed my administrative insight, and was a mistake.' In May 1995, more than a year after the scandal began, the Breast Cancer Prevention Trial began to recruit new participants. The newspapers barely reported the event.

That year, Fisher published a re-analysis of the breast cancer surgery trial. Even with Poisson's fraudulent data removed, the conclusions remained that a lumpectomy was as successful as a radical mastectomy for most patients. The US Government's Office of Research Integrity also completed its investigation, which exonerated Fisher of all charges of scientific misconduct. The report's most damning comment, such as it was, was that the failure to report the misconduct 'contributed in a material way to the uncertainty of the scientific community and in the general public about the validity of important studies'.

In the years since, many doctors have characterised the furore surrounding the Breast Cancer Prevention Trial as emblematic of the media's failure to communicate the subtleties of science; although the investigation of the fraud could have been better managed, newspaper response was disproportionately fierce. 'The whole Kafqaesque episode seems absurd, but also nasty,' wrote twenty luminaries in 1997, in the *Control Clinical Trials*. More importantly, the newspaper frenzy had failed to map the contours of risk for women who were faced with the choice of the two surgical techniques or who were considering taking part in the prevention trial.

After being exonerated, Bernard Fisher was reinstated at the helm of the Breast Cancer Prevention Trial. However, in April 1998 he made the decision to end the trial prematurely: it had been so successful, he said, that it would be unethical to continue to give some of the women the placebo when they ought to be benefiting from tamoxifen. British doctors complained that the results were not nearly clear enough to justify a cessation of the trial. In New Jersey, Renee Rauch, for one, was pleased when she discovered that she had, indeed, been taking the drug and not the placebo, and said that she believed it had helped her keep breast cancer away. Her sister, who had had mammograms throughout her forties, remained confident that her decision had also been correct. Almost a decade on, neither of them have any signs of breast cancer.

'This is an extremely emotional experience for me, probably the most emotional of my entire career,' Fisher told a Washington press conference. The results were that thirty-six women in every thousand who had been taking the placebo had developed breast cancer, compared to only about eighteen and a half per thousand in the group taking tamoxifen. That computed to a 49 per cent reduction in the risk of developing the invasive strain of the disease. In addition, about four fewer women per thousand had suffered complex bone fractures. 'It is the first time in history,' said Fisher, 'that we have evidence that breast cancer can not only be treated but also prevented.'

Yet Cindy Pearson and Adriane Fugh-Berman at the National Women's Health Network, who had sat through the same press conference, interpreted the results in an entirely different way. As they thumbed through the press release, they began to add up the additional illnesses suffered by the women who had taken tamoxifen – illnesses that were far more prevalent than in those who had taken the placebo. About eight more women per thousand had suffered from endometrial cancer during the five years of the trial. And whereas 71 of the 6,599 women taking tamoxifen had suffered 'vascular events' ranging from stroke to deep-vein thrombosis, only 62 of those taking the placebo had suffered the same kind of illnesses. Similarly, 574 women taking tamoxifen had developed cataracts, whereas only 504 of those on the placebo had developed the eye condition. When Fisher published the full results later that year, he was able to show that many of these conditions were not fatal, but they nonetheless provided an unsettling and partial counterbalance to the optimism of the trial's announcement.

In the years since, the idea of using tamoxifen as a preventative for breast cancer in healthy women has remained controversial. Other studies have presented slightly different balances of risk and benefit, and the partisans on both sides have repeatedly returned to the argument. For women who fear that they might develop breast cancer because of a family history of the disease and are contemplating taking tamoxifen to reduce this risk, this ongoing debate makes their decision all the more complex and emotional.

To put oneself at risk in the hope of extending life will become a dilemma that more and more of us will have to face, because in the future medical strategies of prevention and early detection – such as screening or the prescribing of drugs – will play an increasingly important part in cancer medicine. The great breast cancer debates of the 1990s are illustrative of how imperfectly our societies deal with these difficult choices. Across Europe, the debates have been no less partial, incomplete and protracted. The failure to address properly the subtle equations of risks and benefits, therefore, bodes ill for the future: we will be asked to make these decisions but without being given the tools to do so.

§

While reading the articles and books about prevention, I stumbled across a fact that made the questions more pointedly relevant to my own life. In 1993, four doctors at the Wayne

State University School of Medicine, in Detroit, Michigan, had carried out biopsies on young male patients who had no history of prostate cancer. Ten per cent of the men that were in their twenties had undergone changes in their cells that were the first step towards prostate cancer. A quarter of the men that were in their thirties had small clusters of cells that were cancerous.

It meant there was a strong possibility that the precursors of cancer were already inside me. Surrounded by the fear of Dad's cancer, I asked whether I should have some kind of prostate biopsy. But doctors advised me that it would be not only futile but risky – the side effects of biopsies are infections. Moreover, there would be little benefit to me as what might be detected would not necessarily threaten my life, and would be unlikely to do so before my fifties; I was only 36. And the only available prostate cancer screening technology is notoriously unreliable.

It left me with a conundrum. Because when I am older, and the risks of cancer are much greater, and perhaps a doctor has discovered some kind of genetic predisposition within me, or perhaps technology will have become much more precise, then I will be avidly screened for prostate cancer. Until then I will be torn. On the one hand, I understand the logic of those doctors who warn that some current screening regimes for younger people are based on too little scientific evidence, and that there are risks as well as benefits. And on the other I have a belief, founded on some evidence, that some kind of medical intervention must be beneficial, that screening might just pick up something that would otherwise be fatal.

So I do not know when the point will come when I go for my first screen; nor do I entirely understand the criteria by which I will make the decision; will I diligently study the numbers and weigh the odds, or will I reach a point where fear will overcome me and I will be screened in the hope of reassurance?

Targeting Genes:
'my patients made me a crusader'

B UD ROMINE went for a routine medical check-up in September 1994. He had just turned 65 and it was a requirement of his insurers although he showed no symptoms of any disease. The doctor listened to his heart, tested his reflexes and took his blood – the tests would take twenty-four hours to complete. Healthy individuals have between 5,000 and 10,000 white blood cells in each cubic millimetre of blood, but the following day, the doctor phoned Romine up to explain that he had a white blood cell count of 76,000. The most likely cause was leukaemia.

Until then, Romine had appeared to be perfectly healthy. He played golf two or three times a week and he fished the small river at the back of his house in Tillamook, Oregon. Having spent a lifetime as a conductor on the rural lines of the Southern Pacific Railroad, he was relishing his retirement. A video of him taken just a few weeks before the medical appointment shows more than forty family members surrounding him at his birthday party. Portly and holding a bottle of beer, he is overcome and speechless. The tears roll and, though he holds his hands to his eyes, he is unable to stop them. Later in the afternoon, he plays Erroll Garner's jazz standard, 'Misty', on the baby grand piano in the living room.

A day after the results, Romine was lying on his front in a local hospital. A large needle was pushed through his skin and into the hip bone, and Romine felt an immense, grating pain. The bone marrow cells that were extracted were misshapen and oversized, confirming the diagnosis of chronic myeloid leukaemia (CML). Within a week, his white blood count had risen to 124,000, making him tired and breathless and enlarging his spleen. The doctors told him that the prognosis was bleak. For a few years he would live more or less normally with the chronic condition; then billions of white blood cells would overrun his body, gumming up the normal mechanisms like honey in an engine, and within five years he would be dead. 'It knocks you like a loop. It hits you like a blockbuster. It's a death sentence,' remembers Bud. 'It's awfully hard to accept that you only have a few years to go.' Like the low, close clouds that roll across Tillamook from the nearby Oregon shore, a depression enveloped him.

Within days, Romine began taking hydroxyurea, which scythed away the white cells in the blood. In the short term, this allowed Romine to function healthily, his white blood cell count falling to the normal range. This drug did not, however, attack the roots of the disease: the blood-manufacturing cells located in the bone marrow remained, slowly swelling in numbers. Eventually, they would produce more white cells than the hydroxyurea would be able to kill, at which point death would be inevitable.

One other drug promised some hope, interferon, which Romine began taking late in 1994. As well as controlling the numbers of white blood cells, it also killed some of those in the bone marrow, with a slim chance of complete remission. So, each day, Romine injected himself and then battled the side effects, which felt like a continuous bout of very bad flu. 'Just to come out of the bedroom,' he remembers, 'was a hard day's work.' On good days he sat on his porch drifting in and out of sleep, staring at the river. He didn't have the energy or concentration to play the piano any more, and he no longer cherished the future. He could only think one day at a time. Though he had once thought he would live into his eighties, like his father, now he knew that death was not far away.

❧

Dad's inexorable decline, his imminent death, eleven months after surgery, was difficult to grasp. He lay on the bed. I sat in a high-backed hospital chair. For whatever reason we talked less about the past. I showed him photographs of the house that my girlfriend, Andrea, and I were renovating. But he had little interest in a place he would never be able to visit. I talked about foreign places, but he knew he would never travel again. I was desperate to engage him, but I found it difficult to understand the mind of a man who was contemplating his last few days in our world.

Mum's concerns also diverged from ours. Sleepless and harried, she wanted him to be released from hospital to a hospice. She was irritated by the ward's nightly comings and goings, the buzz of the equipment, the moans of the other patients, and the understaffing. Having seen her father die in the cacophony of a hospital ward, she thought it was no place for a man's final breath. Yet the doctors were worried that Dad might not be sufficiently healthy to be moved. Nor was a hospice bed immediately available. Nonetheless, Mum began to ask for a hospice bed for the last days of her husband.

By contrast, Dad's interests were no longer the realities of his health and treatment. Rather, he had a paranoid concern that his granddaughter no longer wished him to read bedtime stories to her. Again and again he mentioned it. That he had become so worried over such a small thing, we thought, was a sign that he might be losing his mind, or perhaps that he was desperate to clutch at an experience that he was leaving behind. So Jessica was persuaded, and Dad sat on his hospital bed in his pyjamas and dressing gown, with one hand holding the book and the other around his granddaughter. Though he could barely gather the strength to stop *The Lion, the Witch and the Wardrobe* from shaking, he battled through its closing chapters, while Jessica swung her legs backwards and forwards.

♊

In the summer of 1993, Dr Brian Druker moved from the Dana-Farber Institute in Boston to the Oregon Health Sciences University in Portland in order to establish his own laboratory to study chronic myeloid leukaemia (CML), the disease that would afflict Bud Romine within the year. Druker was 38 and had an easy way with patients, remembering their families, sharing a chuckle, calming their fears and, where appropriate, assertively offering hope. For an unusually tall, thin man, he somehow managed to appear small and humble in front of them.

Yet it was the laboratory that held him in thrall, with such commitment that he had little time for much of a life outside science. Although his diffident manner made him appear a little uncertain, he strongly believed that he was on the cusp of a revolution in cancer treatment. After 150 years of trying, scientists were at last beginning to sketch out the mechanisms of cancers, of how healthy cells turned malignant. They were drawing up detailed blueprints of exactly which parts of cellular machinery became damaged, and Druker was hoping to use this new knowledge to fix the broken parts of the cancer cell. This approach would be profoundly different from previous cancer treatments, insofar as radiation and chemotherapy worked more or less, but doctors did not understand exactly how they affected the impenetrable black box of the cancer cell. Druker's hope was to create a so-called targeted treatment. He had chosen CML because its mechanism had been described in much greater detail, and with a greater degree of certainty, than any other cancer.

The first two cases of chronic myeloid leukaemia in the medical literature were that of Marie Straide, described by Rudolf Virchow, and a similar case detailed by the Scottish doctor John Hughes Bennett, both published in 1845. Virchow went on to coin the term 'leukaemia' and identify that it was the proliferation of white blood cells that caused the symptoms.

In 1960, two researchers from Philadelphia discovered that over-abundant cells in the bone marrow and blood of CML patients usually contained a shortened twenty-second chromosome, which became known as the 'Philadelphia chromosome'. In 1973, another scientist showed that, in fact, one end of the twenty-second chromosome in the cancerous cells had become detached and fused itself to the end of the ninth chromosome, while the shorter end of the ninth had fixed itself to the twenty-second.

It was unclear why exactly this transposition would create a cancer, until Robert Weinberg and his colleagues discovered, in 1982, that a faulty gene can instruct cells to divide uncontrollably. Within a few years, it was determined that the Philadelphia chromosome contains such a malignant gene. The gene that is created consists of the head of one existing gene and the tail of another, so scientists describe it as 'chimeric', like the mythic beast that was half lion, half goat. Its effect is to send an incessant signal for the cell to divide.

It is as if a single chromosome is a typed-out manual. Each cell has complete copies of twenty-three pairs of manuals. However the Philadelphia chromosome occurs when some of the pages of two of these manuals become detached, and these loose pages are attached to the backs of the wrong manuals. For the most part, this does not affect the harmonious functioning of the cell, as the paragraphs and sentences in the middle sections remain unchanged by the transposition. But where the first half of one manual meets the pages from another, then a new sentence is created with a very different meaning: a false signal to divide.

By the time Druker arrived in Oregon in 1993, he understood that the false signal was created by molecules of a protein manufactured by the chimeric gene. In a diseased cell, these loitered harmlessly around, until they reach a cellular switch and triggered the process of cell division. Druker's belief was that it would be possible to prevent only these rogue proteins from ever reaching the switch. And unlike other cancers where the constant cell division was caused by a series of genes, CML appeared to be comparatively simple, in that only one gene and one protein were involved. Druker reasoned, therefore, that here the principle would be proved that it was possible to correct cancer's genetic mistakes. Such an innovation would be of profound importance, because it would demonstrate the worth of searching for other treatments that targeted just the genetic errors of other, more complicated cancers.

To paralyse the rogue protein, Druker began looking for a molecule that would cling on to it within the diseased cell, thus preventing the triggering of the switch of cell division. The difficulty was in finding a molecule that would not similarly immobilise the hundreds of thousands of proteins that were required for the normal functioning of a cell. His first call was Nick Lydon at a Swiss drug company called Ciba-Geigy.

Since 1985, Lydon had been working in a team to synthesise a whole collection of such molecules. But his strategy was much broader than Druker's. Ciba-Geigy were hoping to discover drugs that might treat the commoner cancers, such as those of the breast and lung. However, in the late 1980s, Druker had met Lydon and suggested that he should focus on CML because the disease appeared so much simpler. Thereafter, Lydon had spent months perfecting a laboratory technique to test new molecules against the CML protein. After Lydon had created a way to measure the molecules' effectiveness, a chemist called Jürg Zimmerman spent two years engineering molecules that paralysed the protein. Rather like a meticulous craftsman, Zimmerman chiselled and honed his molecules so that they would lock on to the cancerous protein like a spanner on a bolt – without erroneously fitting on to any of the other cells' healthy proteins.

In October 1993, Lydon sent Druker five of his best molecules. Druker began to test them on blood that he had recently drawn from his patients. The molecule that Lydon most favoured, however, killed too many healthy cells which jostled with the diseased cells in the test tubes. Three others had no effect at all. But the drug number CGP57148 killed only leukaemic cells. 'It just looked perfect,' Druker remembers thinking. For more than a year, Druker experimented, trying different quantities of the drug with leukaemia cells drawn from a range of patients. In parallel, Ciba-Geigy began testing to make sure that the drug wasn't toxic to animals. With each success, Druker became more excited.

By the beginning of 1995, Druker's accumulated results were ready for publication. Although he thought them to be historically important, the editor of one prestigious journal declined them because there was no evidence that the drug cured the disease in animals; another said they contained no scientific innovation. Eventually they were published in *Nature Medicine*, in April 1996. When his local paper picked up the story, Druker boasted that a clinical trial on patients would begin by the end of the year, as thus far the drug had only been tried on cells in test tubes and animals. Druker was hopeful that his findings would have profound implications: 'If it's working here [in the lab], then it's likely to work for more common cancers like lung cancer, breast cancer and colon cancer,' he told the *Seattle Times*.

The Oregonian landed on Bud Romine's doorstep on 30 April. Brian Druker's face stared out of the front page. It was eighteen months since Romine had been diagnosed. 'We didn't have any hope until then,' remembered his wife, Yvonne. 'But from then on Bud had the will power to keep going, not to quit. He was a strong man.' They wrote to Druker, who invited them to Portland for blood and bone marrow tests. During the following months, over repeated visits, Yvonne and Bud came to see Druker almost as a member of their family.

However, at just the moment when Druker was feeling optimistic about his results, dogs receiving the drug intravenously at Ciba-Geigy were developing blood clots. As a result, Druker's clinical trial on humans was postponed indefinitely. 'I went into a bout of depression,' remembered Druker. 'The rug was pulled out from under me.'

Yet Druker held on to a narrow thread of hope and became more determined that this potentially innovative drug would at least be tested on patients. So, in the summer of 1996, he travelled to Switzerland in an effort to persuade the drug company's scientists and managers to agree to a patient trial. Even before he could properly lay out his argument, he was told that the drug had created liver problems in animals that were taking it orally, which provided yet another obstacle to testing it on patients. At the same time, Ciba-Geigy had merged with Sandoz to become one of the world's largest drug companies, with the new name of Novartis. The combination of the drug's toxicity and corporate restructuring led Druker to feel that the drug – now renamed STI-571 – was 'on the chopping block', especially as Nick Lydon, one of the drug's champions within the company, had recently moved on. Fearing that STI-571 was about to be quietly shelved, Druker returned to Oregon.

§

Four weeks after arriving in hospital, Dad was ready to move to St Mary's Hospice. By now, Dad could no longer stand

and barely had the strength to manoeuvre in bed. Even relieving himself required a hoist and three nurses. The morning of the move, he was sweating profusely, and in pain. Although I could not be there, I was told that his face rippled with anguish and was devoid of colour. He thought that this was going to be his last day alive. But he was lifted into an ambulance and driven the short distance to the hospice. There he began to relax, and Mum and his sister settled him into his new room.

Until I was eleven, on my way to and from school I walked past the enormous white-fronted house that had become the hospice. My friends and I called it the haunted house. The hospice had opened in 1979, as part of the broader hospice movement that had begun in England a decade before when a nurse called Cicely Saunders opened St Christopher's in the London suburb of Sydenham. Having witnessed the deaths of those that she loved, she had observed that 'as the body becomes weaker, so the spirit becomes stronger'. She believed that towards the end of life it was more important to deal with the patient's pain and improve their sense of well-being than attempt yet more clinical interventions.

When I approached the building for the first time, my mind full of memories of childhood, I feared that it would be a house of pain and death, that the ghosts we had once feared had returned in different clothes. But St Mary's was bright, the staff were cheerful and, compared to the frantic atmosphere that had pervaded the dark Victorian hospital, it was calm and peaceful. Rather than in a busy ward, Dad was in a large room by himself. It was the middle of March; the first bright days of spring, shafts of sunlight cut through the room's french windows. Beyond them was a beautiful garden of meandering paths and carefully planted borders. The doctors at the hospice had also calibrated his drug dosage, so he no longer dropped glasses or dozed off. Nor was he ever in pain. There were many more staff and, through his suffering, he made a concerted effort to learn their names and to charm them, and told us little stories of their lives and aspirations.

Although he was nearer death, his mind seemed clearer. He was sprightly, and cracked jokes. The sparkle had returned to his eyes. I would sit in the large armchair in his room, and for the first time since he had left home I would stay up late with him, talking about my week and drinking red wine with him. Dark and late, these nights were reminiscent of the times we had spent together before his illness. When I left, the nurses told me they'd switch off his light a little later.

ॐ

By the autumn of 1996, Brian Druker was losing hope that the drug STI-571 would ever be tested on patients. In his own clinic, he was seeing patients dying, any one of whom could have been testing the drug. He still remembers those that could not wait: Lothar Kaul, an Internet entrepreneur who died in his thirties; Deana Honstein, a retail sales clerk from Portland who died in her twenties. He was treating others with hydroxyurea and interferon, but they were declining irrevocably. 'It was the patients,' he explained, 'that turned me from a researcher into a crusader.' At the same time, Druker secured an annual $100,000 grant from the Leukemia and Lymphoma Society to proceed with the research.

Inside Novartis, Alex Matter, the then head of oncology drug development, was struggling to justify why the drug was important. Not only did the drug appear to be toxic, but, remembers Matter, a marketing assessment had been carried out that showed that 'we were out of our minds trying to develop the drug … this was a no go'. One problem was that there were only about 10,000 patients in Europe and America who became ill with CML each year (compared with the tens of millions of patients, for instance, with type 2 diabetes), too few to guarantee a profit. Another was the historically poor hit-rate of drug development. Having spent his life working for the Swiss and French pharmaceutical industries, Matter understood that many drugs never make it to market, even after enormous investment. He had witnessed drugs that passed through extensive testing in the laboratory, on animals, and then through three phases of trials on patients, only to fail at the final regulatory hurdle, or because an unforeseen side effect became evident. Even successful drugs were often only marginally more effective than their antecedents or were suitable only for a small portion of the patient community. So even if STI-571 was to prove itself to be an innovative approach to the treatment of cancer, there was little likelihood it would ever make money. As a consequence, it seemed that it was destined to be quietly filed away for ever.

'These were desperate times,' remembers Druker. 'How could I tell patients that the drug company wasn't interested, or that the market wasn't big enough?' Throughout 1997, Druker besieged everyone he knew at Novartis, demanding a trial on patients. When the evidence of toxicity in animals remained an obstacle, he found toxicologists who argued that the side effects in some animal tests should not prevent the development of the drug. 'I had something incredibly promising. I wasn't going to let some marketing person not allow this to go forward. That was unacceptable,' Druker recalls.

Alex Matter was torn between the excitement of the scientific possibilities and the miserable probability that the drug would neither be effective nor make a profit. When in August 1997 no clinical trials had been planned, Druker wrote a letter to Matter outlining why one should go ahead: 'For CML patients this drug offers extreme promise ... The issue is to give the drug a chance.' He also threatened a concerted letter-writing campaign should the drug's development not continue. If Novartis were not prepared to persevere, Druker argued, then they should license it to someone else. 'Brian Druker stiffened our back,' remembers Matter. Putting his doubts to one side and becoming an advocate, he called a meeting with the chief executive, Daniel Vasella, and other top managers. A few days before the meeting, sometime towards the end of 1997, Matter received a piece of good news: STI-571 might block a malignant protein that was active in another rare cancer. Although it was a tentative result, it showed that the market might be a little larger. At the meeting, Matter acknowledged that 'purely rationally speaking on the basis of the toxicity results, on the basis of the marketing analysis, there was not a shred of evidence to go forward on this'. But by equal measure, he believed that it was important to put the principle of targeting just one gene to the test. Not only would it be interesting scientifically, but it would either justify or disprove Matter's principal strategy, as his laboratories were searching for targeted drugs against a range of other, commoner cancers. 'If this drug didn't work, then it was better to know now. Then we should do something else.'

Daniel Vasella had some personal experience of leukaemia, as his sister had died of the disease in 1963 when he was 10 years old: 'Her tragic illness and death had a lasting effect on me. More than any other event, it would inspire me in later life to help others as much as I could.' It was one of the reasons that he agreed to a small-scale Phase I trial consisting of fewer than a hundred patients. Participants would be drawn from Brian Druker's clinic, from the University of California in Los Angeles and from the MD Anderson Hospital in Houston, Texas.

By the time the Phase I trial was being considered, in the spring of 1998, Bud Romine's options were narrowing: after three years on interferon, it was proving ineffectual; and at some point patients usually developed a fatal resistance to hydroxyurea. So Druker chose Romine to be his first patient on the trial, beginning on 25 June 1998. 'There was an overriding sense of excitement,' remembers Druker. 'This was one of the few clinical trials in the history of cancer that made sense: we were targeting the abnormality that was driving the cancer.' At the same time, he was fearful that the drug would fail, or kill Romine, or that the disease would accelerate as other treatments had to be stopped.

After a crew from the local TV station had filmed Romine putting the first STI-571 tablet in his mouth, Druker sat by his bedside. 'I had no idea what the drug was going to do,' he recalls. After an hour, Romine's blood was drawn and analysed. And after each subsequent hour there was relief that nothing catastrophic had occurred. Although the purpose of a Phase I trial is merely to test the safety of a drug at low dosages, there was an outside possibility of a miracle. 'He had survived long enough to take the drug, so our hopes were just as high as they could be,' remembers Yvonne Romine, who was sitting next to her husband, knitting. Each day, Romine took another dose. But day by day, his white blood cell count increased. Without the hydroxyurea or interferon, his body had no defences. Two weeks after starting the trial, white blood cells were so dangerously crowding out the healthy blood that Druker was forced to take Romine off STI-571 and send him home. 'We just didn't feel like doing anything and we didn't feel like seeing anyone,' remembers Yvonne. 'We thought the world had stopped again.' At the end of that summer, Bud and Yvonne travelled to their holiday home in southern California, thinking that it would be their last winter there.

&

Although Dad's mind remained alert, his body was collapsing. There was malignancy throughout his skeleton, and especially in his hips. The rebellious cells were sucking out the energy and resources that would ordinarily have been used for normal bodily functions, in a process called cachexia. His appetite was declining, and he found it difficult to swallow. In turn, with fewer nutrients entering his body, he was losing even more energy. In addition, his left leg was thin and wasting, as if it were being slowly eaten away by a parasite from the inside.

Nonetheless, Dad still had energy for company. I would sit with him for long hours. He said he even enjoyed listening to me on my mobile phone, because it was his only connection to the outside world. Then he would make fun of my telephone manner. He relayed the anecdotes that his visitors had told him. And he worried about the stress that his illness was placing on Mum.

One Sunday we wheeled his bed into the hospice's conservatory, where we held a family party. His children, sister, wife and various members of the extended family all gathered around his bed. His grandchildren fed him strawberries. He toasted our good health. Throughout it all, Dad resolutely showed neither anger nor fear.

At this point, despite all our disappointments as a family, we were dazzled by the power of hope. Although we saw his body collapsing, we were still convinced that he would continue living. To provide for this we made plans to move him home, and took delivery of a hospital bed so that he would be as comfortable as possible. We even began investigating the possibility of installing a downstairs shower.

❦

In July and August 1998, Brian Druker and his colleagues gave the drug to a few more patients. Three patients were given 50 mg with no adverse effects. Four had 85 mg. Each week, he and his colleagues would have a conference call to discuss the blood tests of each one. One week, desperate for results, they excitedly thought that one patient's white blood cell count was stabilising, only to be disappointed the following week as it climbed again. In fact, they had witnessed the normal fluctuations of the disease, in which the blood count naturally falls for a few days, only to increase shortly afterwards.

Druker yearned for a result, but he was aware that most Phase I trials lead nowhere, so he was also cautious. However, the few patients on 85 mg saw their white blood cell counts stabilise. Then, in October, the white blood cell counts of patients on 140 mg fell dramatically. As the results trickled in, although Druker began to sense that something important might be happening, he still remained wary: despite being a rational scientist, he was also superstitious and feared tempting fate. He also felt that he had slanted the trial so that it would deliver a positive result. 'Essentially, I had been selecting the patients who were likely to do well. I hadn't chosen anybody tough.'

So he chose a very ill patient called Sharon Godfrey, as a genuine test of the power of STI-571. Close to death, she was brittle and scared. For six years, she had put on her Sunday best and travelled the 200 miles to Portland for a series of ever more drastic, and ever more futile treatments: hydroxyurea, interferon, and an initial dose of chemotherapy that almost killed her. Once she had been a cleaner in a doctor's clinic; now she was a patient. She'd cry during Druker's consultations, and he'd steady her with a compassionate arm; she took courage from his belief that hope existed. Late in December 1998, he offered her a place on the trial. He told her about the risks of heart attacks, of strokes, of possible liver complications, of her white blood cells increasing uncontrollably. He also told her about the handful of other patients who seemed to be responding to this new drug. Devoid of other options, she became the thirteenth patient to take the drug. When she began taking the daily dose of 250 mg she had 125,000 white blood cells per cubic millimetre. After three days, the number remained steady. 'I felt an enormous sense of relief because it hadn't gone up any further,' remembers Druker. A week later, the printout read 30,000. Within three weeks, Godfrey's blood count was normal. Perhaps most remarkably, because the drug targeted only the malignant protein, she suffered from few other side effects.

Druker was thrilled but he also knew that many ideas throughout the history of medicine had initially seemed as if they would save lives, only to fade with further clinical practice. 'We didn't know how long it would last, and if it didn't last no one would care,' Druker recalled, fearing that Sharon Godfrey's illness would quickly recur.

In the early spring of 1999, Druker and his colleagues in Texas and California gave 250 mg doses to a few more patients. Their white blood cell counts also fell. And Sharon Godfrey's illness did not return.

By March 1999, Bud Romine's health had declined so much that his wife thought he was near death. 'My blood count was elevated real bad, and I was feeling real bad,' remembers Romine. Returning from his holiday home, he met Druker, who offered him another chance with STI-571 at a higher dose. Druker was optimistic but reluctant to make promises. 'I had to protect patients from unrealistic expectations,' Druker remembers. 'I had to guard against myself, against getting too excited.'

When Romine arrived at the hospital on 29 April, his white blood cell count stood at 31,000. Lethargic and worried, he had dragged himself to the trial because he considered it to be his 'last hope', although he also feared that the drug would be as ineffectual as it had been ten months previously. Rather than just a single capsule, the 300 mg dose was now made up from capsules of a smaller quantity that had been manufactured earlier in the clinical trial. He drank apple juice to wash away their bitterness. By the fourth day of taking the drug, his white blood cell count had already fallen to 24,000. The depression that had followed him for almost five years was lifting. Two weeks later, the printout read 16,200. 'There was something that was pulling me out of death's door,' remembers Romine. 'It was like a lead weight came off me.' Within three weeks, his white blood cell count was 5,900, just like a healthy person's. 'There was so much joy when it started [to drop],' remembered Yvonne. Bud enthused, 'I was ecstatic. I couldn't believe it.'

Throughout the early summer of 1999, Sharon Godfrey's and Bud Romine's blood counts remained stable, as did those of a small number of other patients who had also taken the drug. Druker pinned on his office walls photographs of his healthier patients cycling, walking and having barbecues as testament to the drug's ability to give new life. Bud Romine was so confident that the effects were lasting that he decided to buy a new pickup truck. In the clinic's waiting room, where previously there was a mood of despondency, there was now a carnival of joy and relief.

STI-571 had proved itself to be at least as good as hydrox-yurea, insofar as it could scythe away the white blood cells. But none of the patients had seen a complete eradication of the bad cells in their bone marrow. As these bone marrow cells manufactured the white blood cells and constantly swelled in numbers, it was possible, therefore, that the disease would simply return after a few optimistic months. Unless the bad cells in the bone marrow were destroyed, then the drug might extend life by a few years but would not be the cure that Druker hoped for.

&

Just over a year before, in March 1998, Suzan McNamara, a carefree 31-year-old, had been diagnosed with CML, chronic myeloid leukaemia. She worked as a book-keeper in a small business in Montreal, Quebec, while taking an evening degree course in ecology. But the diagnosis had destroyed her: 'I felt my soul leave my body. I had had so many dreams. How could I die when I hadn't even lived yet?' In the weeks following the news, she was afraid and found it difficult to stop weeping. On one occasion she lost control and ran screaming through the hospital corridors.

Like Bud Romine, she was prescribed hydroxyurea. Then

she began a course of interferon. Having decided that she would do anything to beat the disease, she took an enormous dose, one that her doctor told her would 'knock out a football player'. She lost weight and looked ill. She didn't like people looking at her, and would wear layers of clothes to disguise her thinness. 'I knew I had to eat, I was wasting away. But I had no appetite and dreaded eating. I would sit in front of my food and cry.'

By the spring of 1999, it was apparent that the interferon was failing to cull the cells that manufactured white blood cells in her bone marrow, so in time her disease would certainly return. To prevent this, her doctors recommended a bone marrow transplant. For a young woman, they said, it was the only genuine cure available, the only route to old age. But she was uncertain, because half the patients who embarked on this course had no prospect of long-term survival. The problem was that the body's immune system first had to be turned off so that bone marrow would not be rejected, but this also made the body vulnerable to fatal infection. Who would board an airliner, she thought, that had a 50 per cent chance of crashing? But the only other choice was the nightmare of the disease. 'It was such a hard decision; it was like deciding on your life.' Eventually, she declined, believing that 'something else is going to happen'.

Suzan McNamara first heard about STI-571 on an Internet support group, in the spring of 1999. The support group filled her life, with messages from patients around the world and scraps of information from their consultations. Brian Druker also read the same message board and realised that news that he had communicated to some of his patients in the morning would be read by CML sufferers that evening. It was a network of support and activism unlike anything that had come before.

Suzan McNamara printed out the information on STI-571 and took it to her doctor, who patiently explained that most Phase I trials came to nothing, and that a few good early cases would probably be overshadowed by other problems. In any case, she would not be eligible for the trial as her existing drugs had not yet failed completely. Without the hope of STI-571, she didn't know how long she would be able to cope with more interferon: 'After a year, my body couldn't take it any more. Just physically, mentally you start to think that death is better than this, this is not living. I was beginning to reach that point.'

☙

At the end of June 1999, Novartis convened a meeting in Bordeaux to discuss the progress of the trial. Just as Druker was leaving, his colleague from UCLA, Charles Sawyers, told him the news that one of the Californian trial patients, a retired accountant called Ellen Froyd, had had a complete bone marrow response, meaning that no cells with the Philadelphia chromosome were detectable. With very few side effects, billions of malignant bone marrow cells, which had been producing enormous numbers of white blood cells, had been killed off. STI-571 was now not only better than other treatments but also a fundamentally different kind of drug, one that could destroy the roots of the disease.

Druker's excitement, however, was tempered by bad news from Novartis: the company was running out of the drug, as only what was described as a 'lab-scale' quantity had been produced. Yet with the drug's growing success, patients around the world were already clamouring to become participants in the trial. And it was important to begin the next phase of the trial as soon as possible. Fifty kilograms was needed within a few months, and another five hundred by the beginning of the following year. 'Yet Novartis said that it would take nine months to fix the drug supply shortage,' said Druker. As a result, hundreds of dying patients would have to forgo this life-saving treatment. 'I didn't understand why they couldn't just put more resources behind it. All they needed was to put a bunch of chemists on making the drug,' said Druker.

Inside Novartis there was, once again, tension. To rush into production would require millions of dollars spent readying the manufacturing plant, testing the processes and procuring the ingredients. Moreover, to build the manufacturing processes at speed would be technically very difficult. As experimental drugs often fail, there were voices within Novartis who counselled caution, to wait for a robust set of results, which would be gathered over a few more months, before gingerly progressing to the next stage. STI-571 was, after all, supported by evidence from fewer than fifty patients treated for just six months, even if these results had been remarkable. To gamble on this drug so early on, therefore, was considered foolhardy by some.

Throughout the summer of 1999, Druker remained demoralised by what he perceived to be the reluctance of Novartis to push ahead. He spoke to everybody he knew in Novartis to persuade them to produce much more STI-571, but found little traction. 'I felt the risks were high,' remembered Daniel Vasella, the CEO of Novartis. 'Though my goal would be to get the drug to people before they died, if the drug was stillborn, critics would hardly give me credit for trying.' Nonetheless, though it still would not be fast enough for many of Druker's patients, he agreed that some preparation should begin in the manufacturing plants in Ringaskiddy, Ireland.

In September 1999, as work was underway at Novartis, Suzan McNamara's white blood cell count continued to rise, as the power of interferon waned. 'It was almost as if my body was so sick from this drug that it collapsed and couldn't take it any more,' she recalled. At the same time, immature mutated cells called 'blasts' began to appear in her blood, a sign that the disease was progressing, that the malignant cells were bursting out of the bone marrow and that death was approaching. To add to her misery, she had fevers. Another toxic chemotherapy drug was prescribed, but the side effects were so intense that she drifted in and out of consciousness for two weeks. 'I was almost comatose, it was horrible.'

During the eighteen months since diagnosis, she had tried each drug in turn and now only one remained: STI-571. Though overcome with despair, she felt a sudden clarity of purpose. 'I had a power surge,' she said. 'I had no other place to go. I had no time to cry. I knew there was something out there that would get me better.' Though sceptical, her doctor tried to secure a place on the trial but was told that there was a waiting list. Frustrated, McNamara emailed Druker directly, begging him for help, explaining that she was a young woman who did not want to die. He responded almost immediately and, a few days later, they spoke on the telephone. He told her about the 'drug supply shortage', and how he had been encouraging Novartis to accelerate production, but he also acknowledged that he was failing. Then he said, 'But maybe as a patient there is something that you can do.' The last words of the conversation echoed long after Suzan McNamara had put down the telephone.

The next day, she posted a message on the CML support group mailing list, asking if they thought an online petition was a good idea. 'It was a plan A,' she thought. 'At least it's a plan; I didn't think it would ever work. But it was something.' When the group responded enthusiastically, Suzan cobbled together some information on STI-571 and created a web-based petition to demand the accelerated manufacture of the drug. Announcing the petition in an email to everyone she knew, she thought that perhaps 200 people would respond. But within a few days many more had signed up. Within three weeks, 3,030 people had enlisted. She asked another activist, Peter Rowbotham, to draft a letter to Daniel Vasella, the CEO of Novartis. Together they wrote, 'We therefore ask for your assurance that everything will be done to produce a sufficient supply of STI-571 to ensure that the trial investigators are not held up in any way.' She printed the names of the petitioners, enclosed the letter and sent the whole package by Fedex on 12 October 1999.

Daniel Vasella had once trained as a doctor, and he liked to think that he brought a clarity of diagnosis and a speed of action to business. 'I did not want huge numbers of patients stalking us at every turn, demanding that we stop lagging behind in producing this drug,' he remembered. Ever since he had been told of the first positive results for STI-571, he had known of the possibility of a 'patient revolt'. Patients, their doctors and supporters were already contacting the company demanding supplies of the drug. Even though some within the company still cautioned against haste, Daniel Vasella realised the speed of production was not fast enough, so he instructed that more resources be used to produce STI-571.

Druker phoned Suzan McNamara on 2 November, her birthday, to explain that her petition had succeeded. He still believes that it was the 'critical factor' in changing Novartis's mind. The community of patients, fighting for their lives, brought together by the Internet, had forced the hand of one of the world's largest pharmaceutical companies.

A week later, McNamara received a letter from the company's head of Clinical Research and Development, which read: 'Novartis has devoted substantial attention to making sufficient quantities of the agent available as soon as possible.' She typed it verbatim into a message for the Internet group, with the subject, 'We got it! We did it!' Soon afterwards, Druker phoned her, to say that a place on the trial would be available within a month. Meanwhile, Novartis swung their enormous corporate might into accelerating the manufacture of the drug. The core ingredients were shipped to Buildings 552 and 553 in Ringaskiddy; some were so harmful to human life that they required special unloading systems. Usually pharmaceutical companies proceed cautiously, testing, scaling up slowly and perfecting the techniques, but Novartis rushed headlong at the problem. 'When a big drug company puts its weight behind a project it is like nothing you could ever imagine. It is one of the most incredible things I had ever seen,' remembers Druker.

The first public announcement about the wonders of STI-571 was made by Druker at the American Society of Haematology meeting in New Orleans, a few weeks later at the beginning of December 1999. Now the global media latched on to the idea of a drug that had demonstrated it was possible to attack cancer at the level of genes. Most newspapers around the world reported the event as signifying a new era of cancer medicine. 'Words can't describe how gratifying this has been for me. I've dreamed of doing something like this since I was a medical student. I've worked on the project for ten years, on this drug for six, and now I get to see it work in patients,' Druker told CNN. That day, Novartis received 2,000 telephone enquiries about the drug.

❧

Ten days after Dad arrived in the hospice, I visited him. Now he could barely sit up. He found it difficult to eat even the smallest of portions. He could only drink through a straw. He seemed sleepy. As his eyelids flickered, I read him a book review in which a politician criticised the memoirs of a spin doctor. Although I wasn't sure he was listening, I read on. Then, to my surprise, he raised his hand and reprimanded me: I had failed to tell him the name of the reviewer, and this very personal critique made little sense to him without it. I told him, and read on.

After that, Dad drifted into sleep. His breathing was rasping and fitful, the sound of his struggle to keep alive. He was not awake when I left.

❧

On the first day of January, the first of the new millennium, Suzan McNamara left Montreal for Portland. She was still so ill that she could hardly climb a flight of stairs. But she remembers that she was happy: 'I thought I am going to live. For the first time throughout the whole disease this was the first time I thought I am going to see my old age now.' Each day that she took STI-571 she found new energy. For five weeks, in a rented apartment, she rediscovered what it meant to be alive. She went to the cinema and drank alcohol. Suddenly food tasted beautiful. 'I felt like I was reborn from that moment on. All of a sudden my life opened up again. It was the most amazing feeling. The most amazing experience of my whole life was when I went there.' When she returned to Montreal a few months later, she changed her degree to molecular biology.

During 2000, Daniel Vasella had continued to drive the corporate machinery of Novartis to rush through the slow drudgery of the regulatory requirements. Crates of documents were delivered to the Food and Drugs Administration, reporting the results of every patient who had taken the drug, the method of production, all the results of the animal tests and the possible dangers; and their inspectors were ushered around manufacturing plants. Although licensing often takes years, on 10 May 2001, Tommy Thompson, the Secretary of Health and Human Services, and Daniel Vasella announced that Glivec, as STI-571 had been branded, had been approved – less than two years after Bud Romine had begun the clinical trial.

As the years have progressed, the characteristics of Glivec have been more clearly delineated. It is not the cure Druker once hoped it would be, as patients do suffer relapses – particularly those who begin the treatment in the accelerated phase or beyond. The reason that the disease returns is that although the drug kills millions of the bone marrow cells with the Philadelphia chromosome, almost always and inevitably just a few remain and these mutate towards resistance.

Despite this, more than 90 per cent of patients taking Glivec have lived for more than four years since they began treatment – something that was thought impossible when Bud Romine took his first dose. Today, Brian Druker and his colleagues are working on other drugs that target the further genetic mutations which send patients into relapse. His hope is that for most patients in the future, a combination of drugs will be able to hold off the disease well into old age.

Glivec, or Gleevec as it is called outside the United States, was an unprecedented success: no cancer drug had saved lives so quickly, with so few side effects. For 150 years, researchers had been dreaming of understanding the mechanisms of cancer and thus being able to treat the problem. Virchow had discovered and promoted the idea that cells were bad seeds. Richard Doll and Wilhelm Hueper had shown that chemicals triggered the disease, and other researchers had shown how cells in contact with carcinogens mutated into cancer. Robert Weinberg and his colleagues had shown that some mutations were as simple as the malfunctioning of a single gene, which could spark cancer on a Petri dish. Since then, many other researchers had mapped out a whole variety of genes, as if they were cogs, levers and pistons in the engines of various cancers. But Glivec showed that it was possible to repair the genetic aberrations precisely. 'It's the same as taking your car to a mechanic,' says Brian Druker, 'and having them work out what part is broken and having them fix the broken part. That's what Glivec has done. And the goal now is to do that with every cancer. Because just like a car, it won't be the same part that breaks every time. Glivec tells us we can do that, what the path is. It's just a matter of getting that done.'

Bud Romine still lives on a country road in Tillamook, Oregon, playing golf once a week, spending his winters in southern California. 'I just love Brian Druker,' he says. And Suzan McNamara is studying for her Ph.D. in drug resistance to leukaemia: 'Now I just live a normal life, taking my drug every day.'

In the twenty-four hours after I read the book review to Dad, he slept for most of the time. Mum came and went. When I phoned to ask if I should visit, she replied that there was little point. In any case, Dad's sister, Helen, was there for support. Mum also told me that he had woken once, and had smiled at her.

The following day, some of his friends sat around his bed and talked. As one of them told a joke, Mum said, Dad smiled. His frailty and wasting meant he was unable to cough properly; his breathing was weak and uneven.

A few minutes past 5 p.m. on Tuesday 25 March 2003, almost a year since he first felt pain, he stopped breathing for ever.

The Clocks of Mortality:
how a cell is damaged

A T THE MOMENT THAT ĐAD DIED, I was doing that most banally insignificant of activities, buying paint to decorate our new home. My sister was crossing the city to be with Mum, unaware that he was gone. Jessica had insisted on going with her. Then almost five years old, she was on the cusp of understanding the difference between a living grandfather and one who, as she later told me, would soon be helping the flowers to grow. My sister arrived at the hospice to discover that Dad's body was still warm. She hugged him. Jessica stood at the threshold of his room, unsure of what to do. I remained 100 miles away; there seemed to be no point in communing with his body now that his mind had stopped working. Had he been alive, I knew he would have ridiculed our sentimentality and the irrationality of spending too much time dealing with the useless, lifeless material that had been his body for seventy-four years.

There was still some doubt over what had caused his death. We wondered whether the doctors had failed him, or if he had succumbed to some hereditary disease. As a doctor, Mum was determined to find out, and asked for a post-mortem. When elderly patients die of cancer, such an investigation is a rarity, as families usually just want to get on with grieving. Nonetheless, she insisted. Overcome by grief, and determined to see his illness through to its medical end, she was even prepared to observe the autopsy. But the pathologist worked alone. The report revealed that there had been a primary tumour of the prostate, as the doctors had suspected. His hip bone had crumbled from a secondary tumour, and there had been another large growth in his liver. In addition, the bone was crumbling away throughout much of Dad's skeleton. By the time he died, the mutated cells had taken over large parts of his body. Death had saved him from further pain.

❦

The macro-pathology at last allowed us to understand what had happened to Dad in the year since he had been diagnosed. But it also raised another question: what had occurred before he felt the pain?

In one sense this was unanswerable, as the sequence of events stretching back over years had never been observed. At the same time, however, monumental research into the genetic mechanisms of cancer had been carried out since the first cancer gene had been isolated twenty years previously. The current view is that cancer occurs because of the relentless degradation of the genes. Throughout life, it is as if each cell is under constant bombardment; the genes of an old person have collected tiny pockmarks, large craters and misplaced chunks – most of which do not normally affect the functions. But some cells accumulate defects in their central systems. In the case of bowel cancer, researchers have revealed a clearly defined sequence of events that lead to malignancy. The first damage to a cell causes it to duplicate into a small benign lump called a polyp; next the cells of the polyp are damaged so that they begin to duplicate more quickly, thus creating a larger lump; after further damage, the lump becomes an invasive and fast-growing cancer.

In prostate cancer, the sequence has not yet been described with such clarity. Yet it is possible to construct a plausible account, based on the latest scientific evidence, of my father's illness.

$\approx$

When I was a child and Dad was in his early forties, he regularly carried me up the Lakeland fells so that I might see the English landscape laid out below. There is one photograph of him, his hair beaten by the wind, holding me atop a drystone wall and pointing out the landmarks below. At that time, his body mostly functioned like a perfectly optimised system; it ingested sugars to provide energy for his limbs, and it fought the infections that I brought home from school. As we climbed higher up Scafell Pike, he breathed harder. As his kidneys sensed a lack of oxygen, they sent hormones to the bone marrow to manufacture blood cells to transport the oxygen. Other cells created the black tufts of hair on the back of his hands, or replaced his stomach lining after a particularly hard night on the town. All the while, millions of cells were dying as well as being born; his skin cells ebbed away after they had outlived their natural life, and his blood cells died when he ceased doing exercise and returned to his sedentary academic job. Whether each cell lived, divided or died was the outcome of the actions of thousands of molecules, the summation of the will of enzymes, hormones and steroids – as if the route of an ocean liner was being determined by the activities of its many passengers.

One day, a cell in his prostate gland began the process of cell division. During the period of its gestation, each of the twenty-two pairs of chromosomes and the Y and X chromosomes had to be accurately duplicated. Their unique patterns, comprising a few billion nucleic-acid building blocks (the As,

Gs, Cs and Ts), had to be copied and perfectly positioned. After six or so hours when the process was complete, the cell bulged somewhat as it now contained two sets of chromosomes. Was the cell ready to be craned apart? This decision would be made by cellular systems that checked the accuracy of the chromosomal duplication, by determining that each nucleic-acid building block was of the right sort, that the patterns were exactly correct. An error would have been detected once in every million or so nucleic acids, and cell division would have been halted and the mistaken building block replaced. If the damage had been irreparable, then the cell would have been quietly sent to its death. But on that particular evening, everything was apparently in order, so Dad's cell divided.

Yet, in fact, in just that single cell an error had been missed by the quality controllers. On chromosome seventeen, something was amiss and it was passed on to the next generation. It happened to be in the middle of a gene called P53, which was normally centrally involved with error checking and quality control during DNA replication. At that time, it made no difference to the cell because there was another copy of P53 on the twin seventeenth chromosome, which continued to function. Yet although there was a functioning quality controller, for some reason the P53 mutation was passed on to yet another generation when the cell divided. Over the years, the progeny of the first cell were often killed off when the error was detected. But equally, when the error was not detected, some survived.

Of course, these particular cells were not unique or alone. In thousands of other cells around the body similar damage occurred, but there was no effect because our cells contain functioning duplicates of almost all genes. No cell was unlucky to have both copies inactive.

❧

As a child, for Sunday lunches – usually after Mum had become upset at the untidiness of the house – we'd often go to a local Italian restaurant. The fractiousness of the family was overcome by the balm of starched linen tablecloths, ageing Italian waiters and sorbet for pudding. My sister and I would order children's portions of spaghetti, while Dad would relish the steak, lamb or venison.

In the hours afterwards, his stomach would break the food down into its constituent parts. Molecules of proteins and fats from the meat would be carried around his body. A particular class of chemicals called heterocyclic amines (HAs), produced by cooking meat at high temperatures, would have been in the charred exterior of his main course, and would also wander around his body, some molecules entering cells. There the HA would damage DNA, but quality-control systems would soon send the cells to their deaths. In other cells, molecules of the HA would bind to detoxifying molecules, which loiter around the cells. The HA molecules would then be unable to attach themselves harmfully elsewhere, and could not damage the cells. Eventually the HA would be dismantled and excreted.

Some of the crucial detoxifying molecules are manufactured by a gene called GSTP1, which sits on the eleventh chromosome. But one day, the GSTP1 genes in one of Dad's cells were damaged – perhaps because of a weakness from an infection; perhaps by some kind of chemical from the air, or naturally occurring in the food Dad ate; or perhaps just by accident, caused by the impossibility of copying the hundreds of millions of nucleic acids accurately. For whatever reason, the safety mechanism of the GSTP1 genes was switched off, and one cell existed without its defensive shield. Unluckily, the GSTP1 damage occurred on both chromosomes, whereas most genetic errors are introduced to only one of a pair. The damage also occurred in one of the cells that had already had a P53 failure – one of the descendants of the cell that had been damaged some years earlier. In fact, unlucky does not begin to characterise the unlikelihood of these bad mutations occurring in the same cell. Even lotteries that have notoriously bad odds have better chances than cellular mutations occurring simultaneously. The trouble is that the number of cells in our bodies is more than a thousand times the population of the earth, so there are bound to be a few cells that are unlucky. This particular cell, in Dad's prostate, was one such. It divided and divided again, meticulously copying mistakes into its progeny.

❦

In the middle of my adolescence, Dad, having failed to persuade me to listen to opera, found common ground with me in the films of Jacques Tati and Woody Allen. We'd go to the local cinema together, where his booming laughter caused the other people in the audience to turn around. I felt I was dying from embarrassment. But at home it was, as ever, his mortality that I feared.

Testosterone, produced in the testes and adrenal glands, is the bond between men. It changes the male body during puberty, and it flows through the adult body every day, playing a part in the constant renewal of bones and stimulating sperm production. For prostate cells, testosterone carries the message that they should divide. When a molecule of testosterone passes through the walls of any prostate cell, it is first transformed into another compound, as if it were a message boy entering the portals of a grand hotel and forced to change into shirt and tie. This new compound binds to another group of proteins, called the androgen receptors. These sit waiting, like some kind of concierge, outside the nucleus. At last, the androgen receptors, receiving testosterone's news, pass into the nucleus and instruct various genes to begin the process of cell duplication.

By the time of my adolescence, when Dad was in his mid fifties, there were a few thousand of his cells, a volume smaller than the head of a pin, that had a non-functioning GSTP1 detoxification system and one defunct P53 gene. Perhaps it was Dad's fondness for an after-dinner cigarillo, or an urban air molecule or part of that burnt kangaroo that he ate at some eccentric dining club that became the next part of his downfall. For on one occasion, a molecule of a carcinogen worked its way around his system and arrived at the prostate. It passed through the walls of the capillary blood vessels and gravitated by chance towards the damaged cells. Without the decoys produced by the GSTP1, the carcinogen passed into the nucleus and damaged the androgen receptor gene. The damage did not prevent the gene producing androgen receptors, but these receptors functioned slightly differently to those in healthy cells, accepting messages from a whole range of other hormones. This resulted in many more instructions for cell division reaching the nucleus, like useless hotel bellhops passing on every piece of foyer gossip as a genuine message. So the cell divided, and divided again at an accelerated rate, the progeny carrying the single P53 error, the failure of the GSTP1 system and the bad androgen receptor.

❧

When I was in my twenties, I used to meet Dad, who was then in his sixties, in London restaurants. We talked over each other excitedly; he about the pamphlets he was printing, me about my television career, both too self-obsessed really to understand the other. Perhaps that was intimacy, the ability to be together but not really listen to each other. After our farewells, I used to watch him amble towards the station, a little unstable on his feet. On each occasion he seemed a little older, the ticking clock of mortality ringing a little louder. I held the gaze until he rounded the corner, just in case that was the last sight I would have of him.

At that time, it was about twenty years since the P53 gene

had mutated in just one cell in his prostate. He wasn't in any sense ill. There were perhaps a few thousand of these cells with three errors, but there was a brake on the speed at which these mutant cells could spread.

These brakes are called telomeres, and they sit at the end of each chromosome. Each telomere is made of a repeating pattern from a single fragment of DNA. At our births, every telomeres section is complete, but each time a cell divides, a fragment of the telomeres is omitted. The result is a second-generation cell that has shorter telomeres than its parents. As the cells divide and divide again over the course of a life, the telomeres sections are progressively whittled down. After twenty, thirty or fifty such cell generations, depending on the length of the original telomeres, there are no more to be copied and, as a result, the cell dies; so the telomeres are the clocks of our mortality. Odd though it might seem, telomeres have survived evolution because they are of benefit to our bodies. Counting down to death, killing off cell generations when they have lived beyond their usefulness, they are one of the body's own defences against cancer; they keep the body's cells young, and they kill bad cells before they can damage the body.

By the time of Dad's sixty-second birthday, many of the multi-mutated cells – with the damage to the P53 gene, the GSTP1 genes and the androgen receptors – were already the offspring of twenty or so generations and so each time they divided they were killed off by the telomeres system. Even as many cells were dividing, others were being killed off, thereby keeping the numbers of rebel cells in check. By the time his sixty-fifth birthday came along, his prostate contained a lump the size of a mustard seed comprising a few hundred thousand of these thrice damaged cells. The risk of further progress towards disease was increased by enormous numbers of them. And so on one day, one of these cells, in the middle of dividing, mistakenly activated a dormant gene that began to manufacture a protein called telomerase. This had the power to rebuild the telomeres in ageing cells, thereby removing the obstacle to speedy multiplication. From this single, four-times mutated cell there were soon a million more.

At about this time, as part of a standard medical check-up, Dad was given a blood test for a protein called prostate specific antigen (PSA), but the lab reported that he had no abnormal levels – about 15 per cent of men with 'normal' PSA will actually have some kind of tumour. All the while, the multi-mutated cells continued to divide. Even then, compared with the malignant tumours that occur in other parts of the body, those in the prostate grow incredibly slowly. On one occasion a cell separated from the prostate floated into the bloodstream and ended up in the stomach. But a prostate cell in the stomach is about as obvious and as unwelcome as a pacifist on a battlefield, so Dad's immune system recognised and destroyed it.

૪

Dad's friends surprised him for his seventieth birthday. Mostly retired professors from fields ranging from chemical weapons to Byronic literature, they were cheery, giving comical, overblown speeches with references that mostly went over my head. But there was a sense of loss as well, because none of them had quite the stamina for staying up late or for getting drunk as they once would have.

By then, Dad's prostate tumour contained a million cells and was the size of a lentil, though he felt no symptoms. In these cells, there was one damaged copy of the P53 gene, the GSTP1 detoxification system was disabled, the androgen receptor was squealing additional signals, and the telomerase was dangerously reconstructing the gene. In other parts of his body, there were other small growths and defects – but none was yet serious.

Each of the cells in the prostate was protected from further damage because the second copy of the P53 gene continued to contribute to the system that controlled the quality of the DNA. But at some point this copy of the gene was also deleted, destroying the principal mechanism for the protection of the genome. When this cell replicated, the quality control system no longer existed; genetic errors proliferated. With each progeny, the genes became more unstable: some lost whole series of brakes on cell division; some quickly became pitted with mistakes and defects. As the numbers multiplied, the cells lived and died by Darwinian selection: those that were most successful at dividing, at commandeering the body's resources and remaining alive, thrived; while the less able died.

With each generation the tumour became more attuned to its environment. Other mutations began to send messages to build blood vessels towards the tumour. Other defects removed the cells' reluctance to expand into otherwise occupied territory. Dad felt nothing. Had anyone done a PSA test, nothing would have been revealed, because, for whatever peculiar reason, Dad's PSA level never rose. Only if a biopsy had been taken might the impending danger of the misshapen, angry cells blooming in his prostate have been seen.

੪

Soon after his seventy-first birthday, Dad and I holed up together in a rural cottage in the South of France. We cooked competitively. I was burdened by wanting to tell him how much I loved and cared for him. I rolled the words around in my mouth, but they never came out. Sitting in shorts, spitting pistachio-nut shells into the undergrowth and talking, we were as close as when he had held me as a child on the drystone wall.

The tumour was the size of the pea and contained hundreds of millions of a great diversity of cells, each descended from the four-time mutated cells but now with various aberrations. The cells were dividing at a greater speed than the surrounding tissue that they were invading.

In the course of this chaos, another gene in one of the damaged cells mutated, which in turn changed hundreds of the regulatory systems that collectively created some parts of the 'identity' of that cell. The damage was akin to a human suffering a massive amnesic shock: the cell no longer knew exactly what kind it was, where it lived, or what it was supposed to do. This particular cell divided and divided, creating a whole species of absent-minded progeny. Without the discipline of this gene, these cells pushed into the surrounding territory. Others were swept away in the increasing blood supply around the cell, and danced off into the rest of the body. The loss of cellular identity meant that these prostate cells had chameleon characteristics, making them invisible to the immune system. One of the bad cells rested on a vertebrae in Dad's neck.

❧

Dad had been an editor of an academic journal as part of his career, and when my first book was being produced, he offered to help. At the age of 73, he came to London and sat on a hard chair in my kitchen, wielding his red pen. For whatever reason I was in a rush. I let him carry on with my work while I went out. He let himself out, and went home. At the moment of greatest threat, I seemed to have lost my fear that each moment might be precious.

As the malignant prostate cell settled in Dad's spine, it released proteins that stimulated the bone cells to divide. These bone cells produced more proteins, which, in turn, stimulated the bad prostate cells to divide. Months before Dad first felt the pain, these multiply damaged cells were spreading slowly through his neck, like the filaments of dry rot through the brickwork of a house. The healthy cells were pushed aside. The closely built structure of the bone was infiltrated by the spongy glandular cells. The structure of the bone began to weaken.

The number of malignant cells was rising exponentially. And while the doubling of a single cell can take twenty generations to produce a tumour the size of a droplet of water, after twenty more generations the tumour would be the size of a grapefruit. Every six months or so, the tumour would double in size. As a mathematician, Dad had always been fascinated by large numbers; as a patient, he both felt and understood their visceral force.

By the time he felt the pain, the seeds of cancer were spreading throughout his body. The surgeon heroically lifted billions of cells out of his neck, and the radiation oncologist killed many millions more a few months later, but it took only a single fast-growing cell for the disease to continue – which it relentlessly did.

☙

Death turned out to be a practical event, one that required project management and negotiation skills: a death certificate had to be procured, funeral directors booked, invitations sent and the wake's menu devised. The most challenging aspect was writing the humanist service, for although Dad had suggested the readings, we had to edit and compile them into a booklet, and then ask his old friends to read or deliver eulogies. The ordinariness of the many tasks contrasted with the loss and remorse that we had all been wrestling with for months. The very concreteness, however, and certainty of those endless lists was a comfort. It was mirrored by the dry language and the cold precision of the typed post-mortem report; and more obliquely by the pile of papers through which I had traced what might have been each molecular step that had led to his tumours. That the cause of the cancer was, to some extent, tangible came as a relief after all those months of waiting.

Epilogue:
the future

CAREFULLY CHOREOGRAPHED BY DAD HIMSELF, the funeral was attended by 200 mourners – a few more than the thirty he had once estimated. Musicians played his favourite pieces. There were readings, and his friends gave speeches. I told the assembled crowd that I loved him; previously, I had only ever been able to express such a feeling in writing. In the days and weeks after his death, I drew solace from the gathering at his funeral, the thought that his grandchildren had been feeding him strawberries almost until the end, and the support of my mother, sister and girlfriend.

There was also consolation to be had in humanity's refusal to capitulate to the disease which had killed him. Angry as I might have been that nothing could have been done for Dad, thousands of scientists and physicians had made enormous efforts over a century and a half to heal him and all those who had suffered. Great men and women had made monumental discoveries, which others had refined and improved. The latest techniques of surgery and radiation therapy had certainly prolonged Dad's life and improved its quality. Twenty years before, the operation that gave him another year of good life would not even have been considered. Similarly, two decades after Mum's first breast cancer diagnosis, she still brims with vitality.

❧

Throughout his illness and the writing of this book, there was a lingering question that I wanted answered: was humanity any better at dealing with this disease than it had been 200 years ago? At first the answer seemed straightforward: Dad's life had been extended, and the techniques were more advanced. But at the same time, I became aware through casual conversation that many people thought that the problem of cancer was getting worse, not least because there are rising rates of incidence. There had also been some critics in the 1980s who had simply argued that we were losing the war against cancer.

One reason there is so much uncertainty is that even the most apparently straightforward statistics are disputed. How long women survive on average after their breast cancer diagnoses would seem, for instance, an incontestable fact. But it is not uncontroversial. The scientific optimists claim that, during the last century, times of survival have been improving: in 1900, as few as 30 per cent of those with localised breast cancer lived beyond five years; by 1950, the survival rate was closer to 80 per cent; and today it is nearer to 98 per cent. However, other researchers argue that these figures mostly demonstrate that medicine is better at detecting breast cancer earlier, so women live longer after their diagnoses but not to an older age.

The rising rates of incidence also do not necessarily point to a growing prevalence of the disease. The numbers of prostate cancers diagnosed, for instance, rose by about 60 per cent in Britain, America and elsewhere during the 1990s. Yet most scientists would agree that there has not been a growing epidemic of the disease; rather, many men who would previously never have been diagnosed have had their cancer identified because of the new technology of the prostate specific antigen test.

Yet there is one way of measuring the cancer problem that is apparently the least open to different interpretations: the so-called age-standardised mortality rate, which allows epidemiologists to compare today's death rates with those of previous generations, while excluding the influence of the increasing age of the population. And by this measurement, for the first time in history, humanity is achieving something in its struggle against cancer – at least in the developed world. Because although cancer death rates were rising quite dramatically throughout the twentieth century, since about 1993 the age-standardised mortality rate of all cancers taken together has been in decline. In America, the rate has decreased by 1.5 per cent a year among men, and by 0.8 per cent a year among women. In Britain, there have been very similar falls. In total, that is about a 10 per cent reduction in deaths from cancer across the decade.

Some specific types of cancer have seen greater decreases. The death rate from breast cancer, for instance, has declined by almost a quarter during the last decade – the result, probably, of treating women after surgery with tamoxifen and chemotherapy, as well as screening women over 50 years old. Tens of thousands of deaths have been averted each year in Europe and America as a result. Similarly, male deaths from lung cancer have been falling in line with the decline of smoking – a reduction of about a quarter of the annual deaths from lung cancer in the UK and a little less of a reduction than this in the US.

Although these declines in cancer deaths may not appear as wholeheartedly successful as the vaccines against polio or antibiotics against infectious diseases, they are a substantial triumph. They are the signs that understanding of the disease is leading to a control of the causes and that medicine is now more effective in intervening once the disease takes hold. For a disease that has proved so intractable, these numbers speak of unprecedented achievements and are a sign of hope.

Of course, there is a counterpoint: some sorts of cancer deaths have continued to increase. Malignant melanoma, a cancer of the skin partly caused by the sun's radiation, is increasing at between 1 and 2 per cent in most western countries. And deaths from cancers of the uterus and certain adult leukaemias are marginally increasing.

How these trends play out in the future, like much else in the highly charged world of cancer politics, remains in dispute. On one side of the argument: Andrew von Eschenbach, the director of the US Government's National Cancer Institute – arguably the most powerful cancer bureaucrat in the world – said in February 2003 that the goal of his institute is to 'eliminate suffering and death from cancer by 2015'. He argues that the continuing revolution in molecular biology will lead to rapid advances in our understanding of the mechanisms of cancer, which in turn will result in a vast array of targeted genetic drugs such as Glivec. In an echo of Nixon's promise, three decades previously, Eschenbach said, 'It is like putting a man on the moon in a decade. We have to make it a reality. I believe we have to do it.'

Holding the opposing view is Samuel Epstein, the emeritus professor of environmental and occupational medicine at the University of Illinois. In his book *Cancer-Gate* (2005) he claims that governments and the National Cancer Institute have failed to tackle environmental pollutants, and that their focus on treatments rather than prevention will fail to reduce the numbers of cancer deaths. Working from the premise that 'cancer is an essentially preventable disease' Epstein's plan of action is for industry and government to control the chemicals in our diet and environment.

Such a polarity of opinion about the future, between scientific optimists and environmental pessimists, has a long history. But in hindsight, neither position has been clearly validated by the current reality. Rather, the last 200 years of cancer medicine reveals a story of jagged, haphazard and erratic incremental progress. And there is every reason, I believe, that this will continue.

This cumulative advance in medicine will lead to profound changes in how cancer is treated in the next few decades. By 2025, writes Karol Sikora, the professor of cancer medicine at the Imperial College of Medicine in London, in a report entitled *Cancer 2025: The Future of Cancer Care*, it 'will be considered a chronic disease, joining conditions such as diabetes, heart diseases and asthma. These conditions impact on the way people live but do not inexorably lead to death.' In this vision, which draws on the views of fifty healthcare professionals, doctors and policy makers, cancer deaths will be pushed further into old age, as the relentless damage to our genomes can be curtailed but not eliminated. Sikora believes that cancers will be detected early in the young and, for the most part, managed by a range of different therapies. The way in which early breast cancer is treated with surgery and then managed with tamoxifen is the model that many doctors believe will be replicated, in slightly different ways, for other cancers.

This measured optimism is more firmly grounded than ever before because of the many recent insights into the genetics of cancer. As doctors learn more about how the disease functions, they will be better able to deal with it. Thus in the future, cancers will be diagnosed long before they are malignant, painful, dangerous or even before they appear. The crude physical diagnostic measures of today – such as the identification of breast lumps or cervical screening – will be replaced by blood tests and imaging technologies that search for malfunctioning cells long before they have become truly dangerous. So patients who are at risk – whether because of age, inheritance or medical history – will have the opportunity to be screened. Already testing for the protein CA125, for instance, appears to detect ovarian cancer some eighteen months before patients would normally notice discomfort caused by the disease. This, it is hoped, will hugely increase the time for medical intervention before the tumour has reached a lethal stage.

The genetic revolution is also radically changing how doctors proceed once a cluster of cells has been detected. For while most cancers are described according to where they are initially discovered, be it the lung, prostate or breast, in the future cancers will be categorised according to exactly which genes are causing the malignancy. Cancers of the lung, for instance, which were once thought to be of a type, will now be classified as a series of different diseases, with separate diagnoses and specific treatments. The most cherished hope of many researchers is that this new molecular knowledge will also lead to the development of targeted drugs, which will function in much the same way that Glivec successfully blocks one particular genetic mutation.

Beyond the field of genetics, scientists are also discovering insights into cancer that can be used during treatment. Already it is possible to inject a patient with a radioactive marker and scan them with an X-ray to measure the leakiness of a tumour's blood capillaries, which may, in turn, determine how receptive that tumour will be to radiation and chemotherapy. Some surgeons believe that bad cells could be marked with phosphorescent chemicals, allowing for more precise excision – in rather eerie, spookily lit operating theatres with surgeons wearing night-vision goggles. And there are nanotechnology machines under development that will be steered to particular parts of a tumour to measure the tumour's susceptibility to radiotherapy.

As diagnostic and treatment methods improve, so, undoubtedly, will preventative strategies. There is already a new drug being tested for reducing the risk of breast cancer; it works like tamoxifen by blocking oestrogen, but is thought to display greater benefits and fewer side effects. Similarly, there is a new vaccine that guards against the virus that causes cervical cancer; this could prevent as many as half a million patients from developing the disease each year across the world. And just as the regulatory leash continues to tighten on the tobacco industry, so it seems increasingly likely that similar pressures will be brought to bear on the food industry and its role in obesity as a cause of cancer.

The upward trajectory may falter. Scientists complain that anti-vivisectionists are making it increasingly difficult, for instance, to carry out animal research in Britain; as most advances in cancer have thus far relied partly on animal experimentation, it is possible that such politicking will slow down discovery. Moreover, scientists are complaining about the increasing burden of regulation, which hampers their work: one told me that he could not freely trade cells and information as he and others once did. There is also always the danger that our own behaviour might eclipse all the benefits brought about by medicine; the obesity epidemic, for instance, might cause a wave of cancers as large as those from smoking.

Progress will also be unevenly distributed. By 2025, it is unlikely that all treatments will be widely available to the 14 million cancer patients who will be diagnosed each year in the developing world. Even in the developed world, progress will benefit the richer segments of our societies to a greater extent than the poorer; already the poorer sections of society tend to smoke more and are less willing to seek medical help. And the expensive treatments of the future will be more easily available to the rich and the vocal.

However, we could accelerate the rate of improvement. More money could be invested in understanding the functioning of the cell: historically, this is the kind of basic research that has laid the foundation for new therapies. In the shorter term, prevention could save many lives. There should be further control of tobacco and greater public education about the risks of sunbathing: beaches in the Mediterranean, Florida and the rest of the world remain full of sunbathers, while in Australia there is much greater awareness of the dangers. Similarly, there could be much more education about diet and greater opportunities for cancer screening.

Although medicine is progressing, public attitudes still lag behind. The disease remains shrouded by taboo. In the years of writing this book and talking casually about the disease, I have seen people shiver as if the devil had walked over their soul; I have seen affable men silently moonwalk away as if I had uttered a stream of invective; others have tilted their head, pursed their lips and emitted a deep sigh; and some have told me that all cancer deaths are long drawn out and nasty.

These attitudes can have a very real effect on patients. The British cancer charity BACUP showed that many employees drop out of the labour market after cancer treatment as a result of the 'isolation, loss of self-esteem, and lack of confidence in their ability to work effectively' because too few organisations offer sufficient support and flexibility. Similarly, there is a body of evidence which suggests that the fear of cancer is making prospective patients reluctant to present their symptoms to doctors, creating a delay that substantially affects survival.

There needs therefore to be a thoroughgoing change in these taboo-shrouded attitudes, a rejection of those opinions rooted in the past, in Galen's physiological melancholy or in the Victorians' fear of the incurable. And equally there has to be reorientation away from the heady optimism that cancer can be cured, and its flipside that a failure to discover the 'magic bullet' is a tragedy for humanity. The trouble with these ideas is that they have little to do with the biological reality of the disease.

This transformation of attitudes ought to begin with how we respond to patients. As the English writer Julia Darling wrote while she was suffering from cancer in 2002 in her poem 'How to Behave with the Ill':

Be direct, say 'How's your cancer?'
Try not to say how well we look

compared to when you met in Safeway's.
Please don't cry, or get emotional,
and say how dreadful it all is.
Also (and this is hard I know)
try not to ignore the ill, or to scurry
past, muttering about a bus, the bank.
Remember that this day might be your last
and that it is a miracle that any of us
stands up, breathes, behaves at all.

We need desperately, therefore, to learn how to talk about cancer, and to regard it no longer as a painful taboo. There is an urgent need to do so, because each of us will one day be touched by the disease, as one in three people will be diagnosed with it within their lifetimes. It is time to understand that cancer is becoming a disease to live with rather than only die from.

❦

A few months after Dad's funeral, my family gathered on the banks of our local canal. As the sun cut through the leaves, the day reminded me of the summers I had spent with Dad at that very spot, painting the small canal boat that we moored there. The university campanile was ringing. Each of us carried a bag with a portion of Dad's ashes. No one spoke.

Then each of us began to scatter our separate bags of ashes. Mum poured them into the reeds. My aunt scared the moorhens as she launched hers on to the glassy surface of the water. My sister spooned them on to the trunks of trees. When eventually I gathered up the courage to touch them, I found his ashes grittier and whiter than I had expected. As they fell through my fingers on to the ground, my shoes were dusted. Calcium, carbon, hydrogen, oxygen and all the elements of the body, now disordered. Not a single filament of DNA remained, nothing that could be termed life.

These same atoms had probably existed at the very moment, tens of millions of years ago, when life itself was being forged, when the first links of DNA were being built into the nuclei of single-celled organisms. The remarkable quality of DNA was that, as new species evolved, so some of the genes built from it were passed on from simple organisms like yeast, to animals and then to humans. That certain genes were so robust and unchanging meant that the lessons of one species could be passed on to another, thereby creating complex organisms over millions of years. Of course, the other countervailing requirement for evolution is that genes are infinitely mutable. The diversity of the whole of the natural world – from each bird's wing, tree's leaf, even Dad's upright posture, his strength and his enquiring mind – depended upon these subtle mutations.

Although it is an essential part of the creation of life, the miraculous process of genetic mutation had also caused Dad's death: the error messages that had instructed the cells of his prostate gland to replicate unchecked had occurred precisely because of DNA's malleability. Cancer's paradox is that its mechanisms are so closely linked to those of life.

My family continued to disperse the ashes. Some remained floating on the surface of the water. A gust of wind took some of them into the air. My family and I stood around, unsure what to do. We had become closer during the previous sixteen months, but we were unable to talk.

Yet the moment extended, and we continued to stare at the ripples, the wind rustling through leaves. Thinking about Dad, I could only hold on to fragments – the stroke of his hands on a beautiful book … the smell of printer's ink and oil … the clatter of the press. I saw us sitting tight together on the roof of our canal boat, chugging through the rainy English countryside; our legs squeezed through the hatch into the warm vibration of the engine room; his hand on the tiller, mine too short to reach.

The ashes began to slip slowly beneath the water, leaving

only a dusting on the surface. I pictured him late at night, across the kitchen table, excitedly telling me about some moment from the past. I remembered the time when he first encouraged me to research the history of cancer. I had thought then that it was to distract me from his pain. Like a willing child, I had been happy to play along. Now, with the ashes returning to nature, I realised that he also would have known that these stories would give me hope. For even when he thought he was dying, he had wanted to teach me about the continuing power of science. He would have wanted to leave me with the belief that, in the future, others like him would live longer because of medicine's successes.

The dusting on the water was replaced by a stillness – as if evolution had reclaimed its own.

My family and I walked back to the car to continue with life.

Acknowledgements

Grateful acknowledgement to the following:

The doctors, scientists and historians who have read all of, or portions of, this book: Professor David Epel, Gitendra Wickremasinghe, Professor Karol Sikora, Professor Henry Harris, Professor John Cairns, Graham Flint, Professor Michael Baum, Professor Mel Greaves, Richard Rettig, Dr Chris Parker, Professor Paolo Domizio, Professor Vivian Nutton, Dr Tim Eisen, Dr Adrian Thomas and Professor Richard Love. Any errors that remain are my own.

Those interviewed for the historical parts of the book: Richard Doll, Bob Weinberg, Chaiho Shih, Michael Wigler, John Cairns, John Bailar III, Charles Weissmann, Mathilde Krim, Bernard Fisher, Allan Campbell, Samuel Broder, James Wolff, Kathy Helzlsouer, Mitch Dowsett, Pat Pilkington, David Henshaw, Cindy Pearson, Helen Cooke, Adriane Fugh-Berman, Heather Goodare, Charles Sawyers and Richard Love.

The Oregon Health & Science University's Cancer Institute: Brian Druker, Rachel Macknight, Tomasz Beer, Grover Bagby and Michael Bagby; to Gloria Stone and Alex Matter from Novartis, and the Glivec patients, Suzan McNamara, Bud Romine, Sharon Godfrey, Judy Orem and Doug Jensen.

Acknowledgements

Those who educated me about the basic principles of cancer: Tim Eisen, Chris Parker, Michael Baum, Karol Sikora, Bill Nelson, Gitendra Wickremasinghe, Paolo Domizio, H. Gilbert Welch and Charlotte Bevan.

The staff of the Wellcome Library, of the science reading room at the British Library and in the Rare Books Department of Columbia University.

My publishers and editors: Andrew Franklin, Daniel Crewe, Penny Daniel and Caroline Pretty at Profile Books, and Elisabeth Schmitz at Grove Atlantic.

The doctors and nurses that cared for Dad, in particular Graham Flint, David Spooner and Vijay Raichura; and all the staff of the University Hospital, Birmingham.

My friends who had the burden of reading the drafts: Tim Tzouliadis, Paul Murphy, Shefali Malhoutra, Stuart Nicholson, Barry Ryan, Gillian du Charme, Charlotte Desai and Leo Hollis. And Andrew Bethell for telling me to write about fathers and sons. Catherine Chesters and Chris Morphet for some great art. And Sasha Vidakovic for his wonderful cover, and his encouragement to print with Dad's type.

This book owes much to the fervour of Patrick Walsh, the best friend and agent an author could have, who tenaciously kept the idea of this book alive and vigorously edited the manuscript in its many many drafts. Also thanks to Emma Parry in New York.

I'd also like to thank my family. My sister Benita for being there during Dad's illness and allowing me to write about her and her children, and to Joe Baker for reading the manuscript. I am very grateful also to Dad's sister Helen Wishart for her comments on the manuscript and for her stoicism and humour during the illness. And to Linnéa Engemann for her putting up with me.

Much of the burden of Dad's illness and then this book fell on Mum. Where others might have turned away from the story that they had experienced, she was a brilliant, prolific and stern critic of the book, while at the same time being infinitely supportive and encouraging. Although this book is dedicated to her husband, it is as much a product of her understanding and education. Thanks, Mum.

Finally, to Andrea Wulf who held my hand through Dad's illness and inspired both him and me to keep talking about history. Her touch is evident on every page of the book, having read the manuscript many times over. But I'm most grateful for the sparkle she brings to my life. Thanks.

Bibliography

General reading

Angier, Natalie, *Natural Obsessions* (Virago, 1988)

Greaves, Mel, *Cancer: The Evolutionary Legacy* (Oxford University Press, 2000)

Kluger, Richard, *Ashes to Ashes* (Alfred A. Knopf, 1996)

Le Fanu, James, *The Rise and Fall of Modern Medicine* (Abacus, 2000)

Lerner, Barron H., *The Breast Cancer Wars* (Oxford University Press, 2001)

Olson, James, *Bathsheba's Breast: Women, Cancer, History* (Johns Hopkins University Press, 2002)

Patterson, James T., *The Dread Disease: Cancer and Modern American Culture* (Harvard University Press, 1987)

Proctor, Robert N., *Cancer Wars: How Politics Shapes What We Know and What We Don't Know* (Basic Books, 1995)

Sontag, Susan, *Illness as Metaphor* (Allen Lane, 1979)

Weinberg, Robert, *One Renegade Cell* (Weidenfeld & Nicolson, 1998)

—, *Racing to the Beginning of the Road* (Bantam Press, 1997)

Welch, H. Gilbert, *Should I Be Tested For Cancer?* (University of California Press, 2004)

From the Ancient Times

American Cancer Society, *Cancer Facts and Figures, 2005* (2005)

Baillie, William, *et al*, 'The Medical Committee of the Society for Investigating the Nature and Cure of Cancer', *Edinburgh Medical and Surgical Journal*, 2 (1806), pp. 382–9

Cancer Research UK, *Cancer Stats Monograph 2004* (2004)

DeMaitre, Luke, 'Medieval Notions of Cancer: Malignancy and Metaphor', *Bulletin of the History of Medicine*, 72 (1998), pp. 609–37

De Moulin, Dr D., 'Historical Notes on Breast Cancer', *Netherlands Journal of Surgery*, 33:4 (1981), p. 206

Franco, G., 'Ramazzini and Workers' Health', *The Lancet*, 354 (1999), pp. 858–61

Jackson, F. I., 'The Strange Case of Ms Elizabeth Trevers who was Affrighted to an Astonishment', *Journal of the Royal Society of Medicine*, 85 (1992), p. 173

Micozzi, M. S., 'Disease in Antiquity: The Case of Cancer', *Archives of Pathology & Laboratory Medicine*, 115 (1991), pp. 838–44

Nutton, Vivian, *Ancient Medicine* (Routledge, 2004)

—, 'Managing a Metaphor: Cancer in Classical Antiquity', *Cancer Topics*, 11 (2000), pp. 6–8

Porter, Roy, *The Greatest Benefit to Mankind* (HarperCollins, 1997)

Reedy, Jeremiah, 'Galen on Cancer and Related Diseases', *Clio Medica*, 10 (1975), pp. 227–38

Retsas, Spyros, *Paleo-Oncology* (Farrand Press, 1986)

Ricci, Ricardo, Rita Lama, Gabriella Di Tota, Arnaldo Capelli and Luigi Capasso, 'Some Considerations about the Incidence of Neoplasms in Human History', *Journal of Paleopathology*, 7 (1995), pp. 5–11

Richardson, Ruth, *Death, Dissection and the Destitute* (Weidenfeld & Nicolson, 2001)

Sappol, Michael, *A Traffic of Dead Bodies* (Princeton University Press, 2002)

Spigelman, M. and P. Bentley, 'Cancer in Ancient Egypt', *Journal of Paleopathology*, 9 (1997), pp. 107–14

Virchow, Rudolph, *Letters to His Parents*, ed. Marie Rabl and trans. L. J. Rather (Science History Publications, 1990)

1831: Surgery

Absolon, Karel B., *Developmental Technology of Gastric Surgery* (Kabel Publishers, 1987)

—, *The Surgeon's Surgeon: Theodor Billroth* (Coronado Press, 1987)

Ayer, Washington, 'An Eye-witness Account of the Discovery of Anaesthesia', in *Milestones in Anaesthesia* (University of Nebraska Press, 1965)

Cameron, Hector, *Reminiscences of Lister* (Jackson, Wylie & Co., 1927)

Cooper, Astley, *Lectures on the Principles and Practice of Surgery* (John Thomas Cox, 1829)

Duncum, Barbara, *The Development of Inhalation Anaesthesia* (Royal Society of Medicine Press, 1994)

Fisher, Richard B., *Joseph Lister 1827–1912* (Macdonald & Jane's, 1977)

Fradin, Dennis, *We Have Conquered Pain* (McElderry Books, 1996)

Godlee, Rickman John, *Lord Lister* (Oxford, 1924)

Guthrie, Douglas, *Lord Lister: His Life and Doctrine* (E. & S. Livingstone, 1949)

Keynes, Geoffrey, *The Life and Works of Sir Astley Cooper* (John Murray, 1922)

The Lancet, 'Guy's Hospital', *The Lancet*, 30–31:2 (1831)

Lister, Joseph, 'A New Method of Treating Compound Fracture, Abscess etc.', *The Lancet*, 16 March 1867, p. 326

—, 'On the Antiseptic Principle in the Practice of Surgery', *British Medical Journal*, 2 (21 September 1867)

Simpson, William, 'Letter', *The Lancet*, 16 April 1831, p. 111

Wolfe, Richard J., *Tarnished Idol: William Thomas Green Morton and the Introduction of Surgical Anesthesia* (Norman Publishing, 2001)

1845: Cells

Ackerknecht, Erwin, *Rudolf Virchow: Doctor, Statesman, Anthropologist* (University of Wisconsin Press, 1953)

Benaroyo, Lazare, 'Rudolf Virchow and the Scientific Approach to Medicine', *Endeavour*, 22:3 (1998), pp. 114–16

Boyd, Byron A., *Rudolf Virchow: The Scientist as Citizen* (Garland Publishing Inc., 1991)

Grunze, Heinz, *History of Clinical Cytology* (G-I-T Verlag E. Giebeler, 1983)

Harris, Henry, *The Birth of the Cell* (Yale University Press, 1998)

Kisch, Bruno, 'Forgotten Leaders in Modern Medicine', *Transactions of the American Philosophical Societies*, 44:2 (1954), p. 227

Lesky, Erna, *The Vienna Medical School of the 19th Century* (Johns Hopkins University Press, 1976)

Long, Esmond, *A History of Pathology* (Bailliere, Tindall & Cox, 1928)

McMenemey, W. H., 'Cellular Pathology, with Special Reference to the Influence of Virchow's Teachings on Medical Thought and Practice', in *Medicine and Science in 1860s* (Wellcome Trust, 1968), pp. 13–43

Parker, A. C., 'On the Discovery of Leukaemia, or Should It Be Leucocythaemia?', *Proceedings of the Royal College of Physicians of Edinburgh*, 20 (1990), pp. 493–501

Rather, Lelland, *A Commentary on the Medical Writings of Rudolf Virchow* (Norman Publishing, 1990)

—, *Disease, Life and Man* (Stanford University Press, 1959)

—, *The Genesis of Cancer* (Johns Hopkins University Press, 1978)

—, 'Virchow's Review of Rokitansky's *Handbuch* in *Preussische Medizinal-Zeitung*, Dec. 1846', *Clio Medica*, 4 (1969), p. 127

Rokitansky, Carl, *A Manual of Pathological Anatomy* (The Sydenham Society, 1854)

Schlumberger, H. G., 'Rudolf Virchow: Revolutionist', *Annals of Medical History*, 4 (1942), pp. 147–53

Virchow, Rudolf, *Cellular Pathology*, ed. L. J. Rather (Dover Publications, 1971)

—, *Cellular Pathology: Editorial*, trans. Lelland Rather, *Disease, Life and Man*, pp. 71–101

—, *A Description and Explanation of the Method of Performing Post-mortem Examinations in the Dead House of the Berlin Charité Hospital* (J. & A. Churchill, 1876)

—, *Letters to His Parents*, ed. Marie Rabl and trans. L. J. Rather (Science History Publications, 1990)

—, 'Standpoints in Scientific Medicine', in *Disease, Life and Man* by Lelland Rather

—, 'Weisses Blut', in *Wissenschaftlichen Medicin von Rudolf Virchow*, (Meidinger Sohn & Comp, 1856), p. 149

1895: Radiation

Béclère, Antoine, 'Le traitement médical des tumeurs hypophysaires, du gigantism et de l'acromégalie par la radiothérapie', *Société Médicale des Hôpitaux*, 19 February 1909, pp. 274ff.

Bernier, Jacques, Eric J. Hall and Amato Giaccia, 'Radiation Oncology: A Century of Achievements', *Nature Reviews*, 4 (2004), p. 737

Clark, Claudia, *Radium Girls: Women and Industrial Health Reform, 1910–1935* (University of North Carolina Press, 1997)

Curie, Eve, *Marie Curie* (Heinemann, 1939)

—, 'One Hundred Years of Radiation Oncology', *Current Radiation Oncology Volume 2*, ed. Thomas Tobias and Thomas Patrick (Edward Arnold, 1996)

—, *Radiological Oncologists: The Unfolding of a Medical Speciality* (Radiology Centennial Inc., 1993)

Curie, Marie, *Pierre Curie* (Dover Publications, 1963)

del Regato, Juan, 'Antoine Béclère', *International Journal of Radiation Oncology Biology, Physics*, 4 (1978), pp. 1069–79

Eisenberg, Ronald, *Radiology: An Illustrated History* (Mosby Year Book, 1992)

Ekirch, Roger, *At Day's Close: Night in Times Past* (Norton, 2005)

Gleaves, Margaret, 'Radium: With a Preliminary Note on Radium Rays in the Treatment of Cancer', *Medical Record*, 7 October 1903

Goldsmith, Barbara, *Obsessive Genius: The Inner World of Marie Curie* (Weidenfeld & Nicolson, 2005)

Hirshberg, Leonard Keene, 'Radium – Discovered by a Woman is a Boon to Her Sex', *Washington Post*, 21 May 1921

Kovarik, Bill, 'Radium Girls', in *Mass Media and Environmental Conflict* (Sage Publications, 2002)

Meloney, Mrs William Brown, 'Introduction', in *Pierre Curie* by Marie Curie (1924)

New York Times, 'Mme. Curie finds America a Marvel', 25 June 1921

—, 'Mme. Curie plans to end all cancers', 12 May 1921

—, 'Power of Roentgen Rays', 4 February 1896

—, 'Radium presented to Madame Curie', 21 May 1921

Nobel Foundation, *Nobel Lectures, Presentation Speeches and Laureates' Biographies: Chemistry 1901–1921* (1966)

Pinell, Patrice, *The Fight Against Cancer in France 1890–1940* (Routledge, 2002)

Quinn, Susan, *Marie Curie: A Life* (Heinemann, 1995)

Reid, Robert, *Marie Curie* (Collins, 1974)

Röntgen, W. C., 'On a New Kind of Ray', *Sitzungsberichte der Würzberger Physic-medic* (1895); trans. Arthur Stanton, *Radiography* (August 1970).

Shaw, George Bernard, *The Doctor's Dilemma* (Constable and Co., 1929)

Washington Post, 'Mme. Curie Drops West Coast Trip', 29 May 1921

1930: Causes

Advisory Committee to the Surgeon General of the Public Health Service, *Smoking and Health* (US Department of Health, Education and Welfare, 1964)

Aronowitz, Robert, 'Balancing Hope, Trust and Truth: Rachel Carson, Her Doctors and Breast Cancer', presented to the History of Cancer Conference, NIH, 2004

Auden, W. H., *Selected Poems*, ed. Edward Mendelson (Faber & Faber, 1979)

Austoker, Joan, *A History of the Imperial Cancer Research Fund 1902–1986* (Oxford University Press, 1988)

The Blue Sheet, 'NIH's Hueper, Authority on Chemical Carcinogens, in Open Revolt', *Blue Street: Drug Research Reports*, 4:17 (13 September 1961)

Brooks, Paul, *The House of Life: Rachel Carson at Work* (Houghton Mifflin, 1972)

Carson, Rachel, *Silent Spring* (Houghton Mifflin, 1962)

Doll, Richard, 'Cohort Studies: History of the Method', in *A History of Epidemiologic Methods and Concepts*, ed. Alfredo Morabia (Birkhäuser Verlag 2004), pp. 152–60

—, 'The First Reports on Smoking and Lung Cancer', in *Ashes to Ashes: The History of Smoking and Health*, ed. by S. Lock, L. A. Reynolds and E. M. Tansey (The Wellcome Trust, 1998)

Doll, Richard and Austin Bradford Hill, 'The Mortality of Doctors in Relation to Their Smoking Habits: A Preliminary Report', *British Medical Journal*, 26 June 1954, p. 4877

—, 'Smoking and Carcinoma of the Lung', *British Medical Journal*, 30 September 1950, p. 4682

Engle, William, 'The Case for the Smoker', *Washington Post*, 9 October 1955, p. 6

Hueper, W. C., *Adventures of a Physician in Occupational Cancer: A Medical Cassandra's Tale*, unpublished manuscript, National Library of Medicine, Bethesda, 1976

—, 'Cancer of the Urinary Bladder in Workers of Chemical Dye Factories and Dyeing Establishments', *Journal of Industrial Hygiene*, 16:5 (1934), p. 255

—, 'Environmental Lung Cancer', *Journal of Medicine in Industry*, 20:2 (1951), p. 49

—, 'Lung Cancer and the Tobacco Smoking Habit', *Industrial Medicine & Surgery*, 23 (1954), pp. 13–19

—, Memorandum Written by Dr Wilhelm Hueper, *Blue Sheet: Drug Research Reports*, 4:17 (13 September 1961)

—, 'Occupational Bladder Cancer', *Proceedings of the Second National Cancer Conference*, p. 361, 1952 (American Cancer Society, 1954)

—, *Occupational Tumors and Allied Diseases* (Charles C. Thomas, 1942)

Kennaway, E. L., 'A Contribution to the Mythology of Cancer Research', *The Lancet*, 26 December 1942, p. 769

—, 'Mythology of Cancer Research, A Letter', *The Lancet*, 8 May 1943, p. 599

The Lancet, 'Medical Research Council's Statement on Tobacco Smoking and Cancer of the Lung', 29 June 1957, p. 134

The Lancet, 'Tobacco and Lung Cancer', 12 August 1950, p. 257

Leopold, Ellen, *A Darker Ribbon: Breast Cancer, Women, and Their Doctors in the Twentieth Century* (Beacon Press, 1999)

New York Times, 'Cancer Aide Urges Tests on Pesticides', 24 July 1963

Parascandola, Mark, 'Two Approaches to Etiology: The Debate over Smoking and Lung Cancer in the 1950s', *Endeavour*, 28:2 (2004)

Proctor, Robert, *The Nazi War on Cancer* (Princeton University Press, 1999)

Reich, Wilhelm, *The Cancer Biopathy* (1948; Vision Press, 1974)

Ross, Walter S., *Crusade: The Official History of the American Cancer Society* (Arbor House, 1987)

Salmon, Cynthia, Mark Knize, Frances Panteleakos, Rebekah Wu, David Nelson and James Felton, 'Minimization of Heterocyclic Amines and Thermal Inactivation of Escherichia Coli in Fried Ground Beef', *Journal of the National Cancer Institute*, 92 (2000), pp. 1773–8

Sellers, Christopher, 'Discovering Environmental Cancer: Wilhelm Hueper, Post-World War II Epidemiology, and the Vanishing Clinician's Eye', *American Journal of Public Health*, 87 (1997), pp. 1824–35

Smith, George Davey, 'Lifestyle, Health, and Health Promotion in Nazi Germany', *British Medical Journal*, 18–25 December 2004, pp. 1424–5

UPI, 'Cancer Official Warns of Pesticide "Dynamite"', *Washington Post*, 24 July 1963, p. A2

UPI, 'Link to Cigarettes Held Unproved', *New York Times*, 27 July 1954, pp. 23, 25

Viorst, Milton, 'Experts Discuss Smoking as Cause of Lung Cancer', *Washington Post*, 21 August 1957, p. C6

Wynder, Ernest L. and Evarts A. Graham, 'Tobacco Smoking as a Possible Etiologic Factor in Bronchiogenic Carcinoma', *Journal of the American Medical Association*, 143:4 (27 May 1950), p. 329

1947: Chemotherapy

Alexander, Stewart, 'Medical Report of the Bari Harbour Mustard Casualties', *Military Surgeon*, 101 (1947), p. 1216

Andrus, E. C. and D. W. Bronk *et al.*, *Advances in Military Medicine* (Little, Brown and Company, 1948)

Brues, Austin, 'The New Emotionalism in Research', *Cancer Research*, 15:6 (July 1955), p. 345

Dameshek, William, 'The Use of Folic Acid Antagonists in the Treatment of Acute and Subacute Leukemia', *Blood*, 4 (1949), p. 168

Farber, Sidney, 'Scope of Chemotherapy in Hodgkins Disease', *Annals of the New York Academy of Science*, 73 (1958), 372–9

—, 'Second Annual David A. Karnofsky Memorial Lecture', *Cancer*, 28 (1971), p. 856

—, 'Some Observations on the Effect of Folic Acid Antagonists on Acute Leukemia and Other Forms of Incurable Cancer', *Blood*, 4 (1949), pp. 160–67

—, Various Letters to Mary Lasker, in the Columbia University Library

Farber, Sidney, Elliott Cutler, James Hawkins, J. Hartwell Harrison, E. Converse Peirce and Gilbert Lenz, 'The Action of Pteroyglutamic Conjugates on Man', *Science*, 19 December 1947, pp. 619–21

Farber, Sidney, Louis Diamond, Robert Mercer, Rober Sylvester and James A. Wolff, 'Temporary Remissions in Acute Leukemia in Children Produced by Folic Acid Antagonist, 4-aminopteroyl-glutamic acid (Aminopterin)', *New England Journal of Medicine*, 239:23 (3 June 1948), pp. 787–93

Farber, Sidney, R. Toch, E. M. Sears and D. Pinkel, 'Advances in Chemotherapy of Cancer in Man', *Advances in Cancer Research*, 4 (1956), pp. 1–71

Frei, Emil, 'The National Cancer Chemotherapy Program', in *Health and Disease: A Reader*, ed. Nick Black, David Boswell, Alastair Gray, Sean Murphy and Jennie Popay (Open University Press, 1984)

Galbraith, J. K., *A Life in Our Times* (Ballantine Books, 1982)

Gellhorn, Alfred, 'Invited Remarks on the Current State of Research in Clinical Chemotherapy', *Cancer Chemotherapy Reports*, 5 (1959), pp. 1–12

Gilman, Alfred, 'The Initial Clinical Trial of Nitrogen Mustard', *American Journal of Surgery*, 105 (1963), pp. 574–8

Goodman, Jordan and Vivien Walsh, *The Story of Taxol: Nature and Politics in the Pursuit of an Anti-cancer Drug* (Cambridge, 2001)

Grealy, Lucy, *Autobiography of a Face* (Houghton Mifflin, 1994)

Lasker, Mary, 'The Unforgettable Character of Dusty Rhoads', *Reader's Digest* (1960)

Laszlo, John, *The Cure of Childhood Leukemia* (Rutgers University Press, 1995)

MacGregor, Alistair, 'The Search for a Chemical Cure for Cancer', *Medical History*, 10 (1966), pp. 374–85

Mercer, Robert D., 'The Team', *Medical and Pediatric Oncology*, 33 (1999), pp. 408–9

New York Times, 'Navy Flying Sick Child', 17 April 1948

New York Times, 'President Proclaims Cancer Month', 26 March 1948

Pochedly, Carl, 'Dr James A. Wolff II First Successful Chemotherapy of Acute Leukemia', *American Journal of Pediatric Hematology*, 6 (1984), pp. 449–54

Ravdin, I. S., 'The Cancer Chemotherapy Program', *Cancer Chemotherapy Reports*, 5 (1959), p. 13

Rettig, Richard, *Cancer Crusade: The Story of the National Cancer Act 1971* (Princeton University Press, 1977)

Ruccione, K. and Fergusson, 'A Living Legend in Pediatric Oncology Nursing: Jean Fergusson', *Journal of Pediatric Oncology Nursing*, 18 (2001), pp. 229–38

Sylvester, Robert, 'Further Reflections', *Medical and Pediatric Oncology*, 33 (1999), p. 408

Wolff, James, 'First Light on the Horizon: The Dawn of Chemotherapy', *Medical and Pediatric Oncology*, 33 (1999), pp. 405–7

—, 'History of Pediatric Oncology', *Pediatric Hematology and Oncology*, 8 (1991), pp. 89–91

Zubrod, C. Gordon, 'Historic Milestones in Curative Chemotherapy', *Seminars in Oncology*, 6 (1979), p. 490

Zubrod, C. Gordon and S. Schepartz, 'The Chemotherapy Program of the National Cancer Institute: History, Analysis and Plans', *Cancer Chemotherapy Reports*, 50 (1966), p. 349

1969: The War on Cancer

Associated Press, 'Scientists Hail Virus Discovery', *Washington Post*, 11 March 1969, p. A11

Auerbach, Stuart, 'Increasing the Odds Against a Rare Bone Cancer', *Washington Post*, 8 March 1974, B1, p. 2

—, 'Institute to Probe Causes of Cancer in "Hot Virus" Lab', *Washington Post*, 9 February 1969, p. 3

—, 'New Virus "Strongly Linked" to Breast Cancer', *Washington Post*, 20 June 1970, p. A3

Bailar, J. C. and E. M. Smith, 'Progress Against Cancer?', *New England Journal of Cancer*, 314 (8 May 1986), pp. 1226–32

Bishop, Jerry, 'The Wrong Way to Fight Cancer', *New York Times*, 16 July 1971, p. 6

Brenner Drew, Elizabeth, 'The Health Syndicate', *Atlantic Monthly* (December 1967), pp. 75–82

Bud, R. F., 'Strategy in American Cancer Research After World War II', *Social Studies in Science*, 8 (1978), pp. 425–59

Burke, Richard, *The Senator: My Years with Senator Kennedy* (St Martin's Press, 1982)

Cantell, Kari, *The Story of Interferon* (World Scientific, 1998)

Cohn, V., 'Scientists Making Copy of Disease-fighting Gene', *Washington Post*, 17 January 1980

Crichton, Michael, *The Andromeda Strain* (Arrow, 1969)

Culliton, Barbara, 'Cancer Advisory Board: Nobody's Rubber Stamp', *Science*, 3 November 1972, p. 479

—, 'Cancer: Select Committee Calls Virus Program Closed Shop', *Science*, 14 December 1973, p. 1110

—, 'Virus Cancer Program: Review Panel Stands by Criticism', *Science*, 12 April 1974, pp. 143–5

Garb, Solomon, *Cure for Cancer: A National Goal* (Springer Publishing Company, 1968)

Gutterman, J. U. and G. R. Blumenschein *et al.*, 'Leukocyte Interferon-Induced Tumour Regression in Human Metastatic Breast Cancer, Multiple Myeloma and Malignant Lymphoma', *Annals of Internal Medicine*, 93 (1980), pp. 399–406

Hall, Stephen S., *A Commotion in the Blood: Life, Death and the Immune System* (Henry Holt & Company, 1997)

Huebner, Robert J. and George J. Todaro, 'Oncogenes of RNA Tumor Viruses as Determinants of Cancer', *Proceedings of the National Academy of Sciences*, 64 (November 1969), pp. 1087–94

Lasker, Mary, 'History of Interferon', Mary Lasker Papers, 1
    December 1978, Columbia University
National Panel of Consultants on the Conquest of Cancer,
    National Program for the Conquest of Cancer, Committee on Labor
    and Public Welfare (United States Senate, 1970)
Panem, Sandra, *The Interferon Crusade* (Brookings Institute, 1984)
Pieters, Toine, 'A Biography of a Wonder Drug', in *100 Years of
    Organized Cancer Research*, ed. Wolfgang Eckart (Georg Theime
    Verlag, 2000)
—, 'Marketing Medicines through Radomised Controlled Trials:
    The Case of Interferon', *British Medical Journal*, 317 (1998), pp.
    231–3
Rettig, Richard, *Cancer Crusade: The Story of the National Cancer Act
    1971* (Princeton University Press, 1977)
Ross, Walter, *Crusade: The Official History of the American Cancer
    Society* (Arbor House, 1987)
Strickland, Stephen P., *Politics, Science and Dread Disease* (Harvard
    University Press, 1972)
Time Magazine, 'The Big IF in Cancer', 31 March 1980
Wade, Nicholas, 'Cloning Gold Rush Turns Basic Biology into
    Big Business', *Science*, 16 May 1980, pp. 688–92
—, 'Race for Human Cancer Virus: Odds Against Houston
    Team Lengthen', *Science*, 24 September 1971, p. 1220
—, 'Special Virus Cancer Program: Travails of a Biological
    Moonshot', *Science*, 24 December 1971, pp. 1306–11
Washington Post, 'Tests Link Some Cancers to Virus, Team of US
    Researchers Report', 5 December 1969, p. A24
Weissmann, Charles, 'Recombinant Interferon – The 20th
    Anniversary', in *Recombinant Protein Drugs*, ed. P. Buckel
    (Birkhauser Verlag, 2001)

1979: Alternatives

Appleyard, Bryan, 'Chaos Creeps up on Science as Two
    Medicines Collide', *Sunday Times*, 9 September 1990
Ausubel, Kenny, *When Healing Becomes a Crime* (Healing Arts Press,
    2000)
Bagenal, F. S., D. F. Easton, E. Harris, C. E. D. Chilvers and
    T. J. McElwain, 'Survival of Patients with Breast Cancer

Attending Bristol Cancer Help Centre', *The Lancet*, 8
September 1990, pp. 606–10

Barrett, Stephen and William Jarvis, *The Health Robbers: A Close
Look at Quackery in America* (Prometheus Books, 1993)

Bodmer, Walter, 'Letter', *The Lancet*, 10 November 1990, p. 1188

Brohn, Penny, *The Bristol Programme* (Century, 1987)

—, *Gentle Giants* (Century, 1986)

Brohn, Penny and Alec Forbes, Bristol Cancer Help Centre
pamphlets, 1982

Bryan, Jenny, 'Ripple of Hope from a Port of Storm', *The
Guardian*, 30 August 1989

Cameron, Ewan and Allan Campbell, 'The Orthomolecular
Treatment of Cancer', *Chem-Bio Interactions* (1974), pp. 285–315

Cameron, Ewan, Allan Campbell and Thomas Jack, 'The
Orthomolecular Treatment of Cancer: Reticulum Cell
Sarcoma: Double Complete Regression', *Chem-Bio Interactions*
(1975), pp. 387–93

Cameron, Ewan and Linus Pauling, 'Supplemental Ascorbate
in the Supportive Treatment of Cancer', *Proceedings of the
National Academy of Sciences*, 73:10 (1976), pp. 3685–9

Campbell, Allan, Thomas Jack and Ewan Cameron, 'Reticulum
Cell Sarcoma: Two Complete "Spontaneous" Regressions, in
Response to High Dose Ascorbic Acid Therapy', *Oncology*, 48
(1991), pp. 495–7

Cooke, Helen, *The Bristol Approach to Living with Cancer* (Robinson,
2003)

Downer, S. M., M. M. Cody, P. McCluskey, P. D. Wilson, S. J.
Arnott, T. A. Lister and M. L. Slevin, 'Pursuit and Practice
of Complementary Therapies by Cancer Patients Receiving
Conventional Treatment', *British Medical Journal*, 9 July 1994,
pp. 86–9

Dye, Lee, 'The Deeply Personal War of Linus Pauling', *Los
Angeles Times*, 2 June 1985, part 6, p. 1

Eisenberg, David, Ronald C. Kessler, Cindy Foster, Frances
E. Norlock, David R. Calkins and Thomas Delbanco,
'Unconventional Medicine in the United States', *New England
Journal of Medicine*, 28 January 1993

Ernst, Edzard, *Complementary Medicine: The Evidence So Far*
(Peninsula Medical School, 2004)

Goodare, Heather, *Fighting Spirit* (Scarlet Press, 1996)

Hager, Thomas, *Force of Nature* (Simon & Schuster, 1995)

Hayes, R. J., P. G. Smith and L. Carpenter, 'Bristol Cancer Help
Centre', *The Lancet*, 10 November 1990, p. 1185

Hill, Chris, 'Cancer Help Study Team Admits Errors', *The
Guardian*, 9 November 1990

Hunt, Liz, 'News of Death Greatly Exaggerated', *The Independent*,
15 November 1993

Illich, Ivan, *Medical Nemesis: The Expropriation of Health* (Calder &
Boyars, 1975)

Laurance, Jeremy, 'Disillusionment, Suspicion, Disaster', *The
Independent*, 11 December 1990

Markle, Gerald and James Petersen, 'Resolution of Laetrile
Controversy: Past Attempts and Future Prospects', in *Scientific
Controversies*, ed. H. Tristram Engelhardt and Arthur L.
Caplan (Cambridge University Press, 1987)

Moss, Ralph, *The Cancer Industry* (Equinox Press, 1980)

Pauling, Linus and Ewan Cameron, *Cancer and Vitamin C: A
Discussion of the Nature, Causes, Prevention and Treatment of Cancer
with Special Reference to the Value of Vitamin C* (Linus Pauling
Institute of Science and Medicine, 1979)

Richards, Evelleen, *Vitamin C and Cancer: Medicine or Politics*
(Macmillan, 1991)

Sheard, T. A. B., 'Bristol Cancer Help Centre', *The Lancet*, 15
September 1990, p. 683

Sherman, Jill, 'Cancer Patients at Holistic Centre "are more
likely to die"', *The Times*, 6 September 1990

Simonton, O., Carl, Stephanie Matthews-Simonton and James
Creighton, *Getting Well Again* (Tarcher, 1978)

The Times, 'Healing Backed by Prince', 17 June 1983

The Times, 'Physician Heal Thyself', 10 August 1983

Walker, Martin J., *Dirty Medicine: Science, Big Business and the Assault
on Natural Health Care* (Slingshot Publications, 1994)

Whorton, James, *Nature Cures: The History of Alternative Medicine in
America* (Oxford University Press, 2002)

1982: Genes

Barbacid, Mariano and Marcos Malumbres, 'RAS Oncogenes: The First 30 years', *Nature Reviews*, 3 (2003), pp. 7–13

Barbacid, Mariano, Simonetta Pulciani, Eugenio Santos, Anne Lauver, Linda Long and Keith Robbins, 'Oncogenes in Human Tumor Cell Lines: Molecular Cloning of a Transforming Gene from Human Bladder Carcinoma Cells', *Proceedings of the National Academy of Sciences*, 79 (1982), pp. 2845–9

Bishop, Michael, 'Cancer: The Rise of the Genetic Paradigm', *Genes and Development*, 9 (1995), pp. 1309–15

Cairns, John, 'The Origin of Human Cancers', *Nature*, 29 January 1981, p. 353

Cooper, Geoffrey, Channing Der and Theodore Krontiris, 'Transforming Genes of Human Bladder and Lung Carcinoma Cell Lines are Homologous to the Ras of Harvey and Kirsten Viruses', *Proceedings of the National Academy of Sciences*, 79 (June 1982), pp. 3637–40

Cooper, Geoffrey and Theodore Krontiris, 'Transforming Activity of Human Tumor DNAs', *Proceedings of the National Academy of Sciences*, 78 (February 1981), pp. 1181–4

Fujimura, Joan, *Crafting Science: A Sociohistory of the Quest for the Genetics of Cancer* (Harvard University Press, 1996)

Goldfarb, M., K. Shimizu, M. Perucho and M. Wigler, 'Isolation and Preliminary Characterization of a Human Transforming Gene from T24 Bladder Carcinoma Cells', *Nature*, 296 (1 April 1982), pp. 404–9

Jones, Steve, *The Language of Genes* (Flamingo, 2000)

Marx, Jean, 'Cancer Cell Genes Linked to Viral oncGenes', *Science*, 216 (14 May 1982), p. 724

—, 'Gene Transfer Yields Cancer Clues', *Science*, 215 (19 February 1982), p. 955

McAuliffe, Sharon and Kathleen McAuliffe, 'The Genetic Assault on Cancer', *New York Times Magazine*, 24 October 1982, p. 39

Morange, Michel, 'From the Regulatory Vision of Cancer to the Oncogene Paradigm, 1975–1985', *Journal of the History of Biology*, 30 (1997), pp. 1–29

Nature, 'Anatomy of a Human Cancer Gene', 300 (11 November 1982)

Nature, 'Two Views of the Causes of Cancer', 239 (5 February 1981), p. 431

Parada, Luis, Clifford Tabbin, Chiaho Shih and Robert Weinberg, 'Human EJ Bladder Carcinoma Oncogene is Homologue of Harvey Sarcoma Virus *Ras* Gene', *Nature*, 297 (10 June 1982), p. 474

Reddy, E. Premkumar, Roberta K. Reynolds, Eugenio Santos and Mariano Barbacid, 'A Point Mutation is Responsible for the Acquisition of Transforming Properties by the T24 Human Bladder Carcinoma Oncogene', *Nature*, 300 (11 November 1982), p. 149

Shih, Chiaho, L. C. Padhy, Mark Murray and Robert Weinberg, 'Tranforming Genes of Carcinomas and Neuroblastomas Introduced Into Mouse Fibroblasts', *Nature*, 290 (19 March 1981), p. 261

Shih, Chiaho, Ben-Zion Shilo, Mitchel Goldfarb, Ann Dannenberg and Robert A. Weinberg, 'Passage of Phenotypes of Chemically Transformed Cells via Transfection of DNA and Chromatin', *Proceedings of the National Academy of Sciences*, 76 (1979), pp. 5714–18

Shih, Chiaho and Robert Weinberg, 'Isolation of a Transforming Sequence from a Human Bladder Carcinoma Cell Line', *Cell*, 29 (1982), pp. 161–9

Tabin, Clifford, S. M. Bradley, C. I. Bargmann, R. A. Weinberg, A. G. Papageorge, E. M. Scolnick, R. Dhar, D. Lowy and E. H. Chang, 'Mechanism of Activation of Human Oncogene', *Nature*, 300 (11 November 1982), p. 143

Weinberg, Robert, 'Fewer and Fewer Oncogenes', *Cell*, 30 (August 1982), pp. 3–4

—, 'A Molecular Basis of Cancer', *Scientific American*, (November 1983), pp. 126–42

—, 'Oncogenes of Human Tumor Cells', *TIBS* (April 1982), pp. 135–6

Wigler, Michael, Kenji Shimzu, Mitch Goldfarb, Yolande Suard, Manuel Perucho, Yen Li, Tohru Kamata, Jim Fermisco, Ed Stavnezer and Jorgen Fogh, 'Three Human Transforming

Genes Are Related to the Viral *Ras* Oncogene', *Proceedings of the National Academy of Sciences*, 80 (April 1983), pp. 2112–16

1992: Prevention
Altman, Lawrence, 'Federal Officials to Review Documents in Breast Cancer Study with Falsified Data', *New York Times*, 27 March 1994, p. 22

Boyd, Robert, 'New Mammogram Report Leaves Women Adrift', *Chicago Tribune*, 24 January 1997

Bush, Trudy and K. J. Helzlsouer, 'Tamoxifen for the Primary Prevention of Breast Cancer: A Review and Critique of the Concept and Trial', *Epidemiologic Reviews* (1993), pp. 233–43

Center for Health Communications, *Report of the Conference on Science, Technology, and the News Media* (Harvard School of Public Health, 1995)

Crewdson, John, 'Fraud in Breast Cancer Study: Doctor Lied on Data for a Decade', *Chicago Tribune*, 13 March 1994, p. 1

Fisher, Bernard, 'A Commentary on Endometrial Cancer Deaths in Tamoxifen-Treated Breast Cancer Patients', *Journal of Clinical Oncology*, 14 (1996), p. 1027

—, 'The Evolution of Paradigms for the Management of Breast Cancer: A Personal Perspective', *Cancer Research*, 52 (1 May 1992), pp. 2371–83

—, 'Highlights of the NSABP Breast Cancer Prevention Trial', *Cancer Control*, 4 (1997)

—, 'Thoughts From a Journey', *Journal of Clinical Oncology*, 11 (December 1993), pp. 2297–305

Fisher, Bernard, Joseph Constantino, Carol Redmond, Edwin Fisher, D. Lawrence Wickerman and Walter M. Cronin, 'Endometrial Cancer in Tamoxifen-Treated Breast Cancer Patients', *Journal of the National Cancer Institute*, 86 (6 April 1994)

Fisher, Bernard, Joseph Constantino, D. Lawrence Wickerman, Carol Redmond, Maureen Kavanah, Walter Cronin, Victor Vogel, Andre Robidoux, Nikolay Dimitrov, James Atkins, Mary Daly, *et al.*, 'Tamoxifen for Prevention of Breast Cancer', *Journal of the National Cancer Institute*, 90 (16 September 1998), p. 1371

Friedman, Sally, 'The Women Who Volunteer for a Cancer-
Prevention Study', *New York Times*, 28 February 1993, p. A1

Fugh-Berman, Adriane, 'Tamoxifen in Healthy Women:
Preventative Health or Preventing Health?', National
Women's Health Network, *Network News* (September/October
1992), p. 3

Fugh-Berman, Adriane and Samuel Epstein, 'Tamoxifen:
Disease Prevention or Disease Substitution', *The Lancet*, 340 (7
November 1992), p. 1143

House of Representatives, Committee on Energy and
Commerce, Subcommittee on Oversight and Investigations:
'Scientific Misconduct in Breast Cancer Research', 13 April
1994

House of Representatives, Human Resources and
Intergovernmental Relations Subcommittee of the
Committee on Government Operations, 'Breast Cancer
Prevention Study: Are Healthy Women Put at Risk by
Federally Funded Research?', 22 October 1992

Jordan, Craig, 'Designer Estrogens', *Scientific American*, 1 October
1998

—, 'Tamoxifen: A Personal Retrospective', *Lancet Oncology*, 1
(2000), pp. 43–9

—, 'Tamoxifen: For the Treatment and Prevention of Breast
Cancer' (PRR, 1999)

Jørgensen, Karsten Juhl and Peter C. Gøtzsche, 'Presentation on
Websites of Possible Benefits and Harms from Screening for
Breast Cancer: Cross Sectional Study', *British Medical Journal*,
17 January 2004, p. 148

Klausner, Richard and Bernard Fisher, 'News Conference to
Discuss a New Study on Effects of Tamoxifen' (FDCH
Political Transcipts, 1998)

Marshall, Eliot, 'Reanalysis Confirms Results of "Tainted"
Study', *Science*, 270 (8 December 1995), p. 1562

—, 'Tamoxifen: Hanging in the Balance', *Science*, 264 (10 June
1994), p. 1534

National Women's Health Network, 'Network Opposes
Tamoxifen Trial', *Network News* (January/February 1991), p. 3

New York Times, 'The Breast Cancer Fabrications', 20 March 1994, p. 16

Olson, James, *Bathsheba's Breast: Women, Cancer & History* (Johns Hopkins University Press, 2002)

Pauker, S. G. and J. P. Kassirer, 'Contentious Screening Decisions – Does the Choice Matter?', *New England Journal of Medicine*, 336 (24 April 1997), p. 1243

Pearson, Cindy, 'Estrogen Without Cancer? Don't Bet Your Life On It', National Women's Health Network, *Network News*, March/April 1998

—, 'Congress Holds Hearing on Tamoxifen Trial', National Women's Health Network, *Network News* (January/February 1993)

—, 'NCI Warns Women on Tamoxifen of Risk of Fatal Uterine Cancer', National Women's Health Network, *Network News*, (March/April 1994)

Peto, Richard, R. Collins, D. Sackett, J. Darbyshire, A. Babiker, M. Buyse, H. Stewart, M. Baum, A. Goldhirsch, G. Bonadonna, P. Valagussa, L. Rutqvist, D. Elbourne, C. Davies, O. Dalesio, M. Parmar, C. Hill, M. Clarke, R. Gray and R. Doll, 'The Trials of Dr. Bernard Fisher: A European Perspective', *Control Clinical Trials* (February 1997), pp. 1–13

Rennie, Drummond, 'Editorial: Breast Cancer How to Handle Misconduct', *Journal of the American Medical Association*, 271 (20 April 1994), p. 1205

Roan, Shari, 'Cancer Prevention Trials Open New Era in Medicine', *Los Angeles Times*, 7 September 1992, p. 1

Sakr, W. A., G. P. Haas, B. F. Cassin, J. E. Pontes and J. D. Crissman, 'The Frequency of Carcinoma and Intraepithelial Neoplasia of the Prostate in Young Male Patients', *Journal of Urology* (August 1993), pp. 379–85

—, 'NIH Tightens Clinical Trial Monitoring', *Science*, 264 (22 April 1994), p. 499

—, 'Restating the Risks of Tamoxifen', *Science*, 263 (18 February 1994), p. 910

Wells, Jane, 'Mammography and the Politics of Randomised Controlled Trials', *British Medical Journal*, 317 (31 October 1998), pp. 1224–30

1999: Targeting Genes

Druker, Bryan, Shu Tamura, Elisabeth Buchindunger, Sayuri
Ohno, Gerald Segal, Shane Fannings, Jürg Zimmermann and
Nicholas Lydon, 'Effects of a Selective Inhibitor of the Abl
Tyrosine Kinase on the Growth of Bcr-Abl Positive Cells',
Nature Medicine, 2 (May 1996), p. 561

Hardy, Alexandra, 'Drug May Offer Hope to Adults with
Leukemia', *Seattle Times*, 12 May 1996

Koglin, Oz Hopkins, 'New Drug May Fight Common
Leukemia', *The Oregonian*, 30 April 1996

Vasella, Daniel, *Magic Cancer Bullet* (Harper Business, 2003)

2003: The Clocks of Mortality

Fordyce, C. A., C. M. Heaphy, N. E. Joste, A. Y. Smith, W. C.
Hunt, J. K. Griffith, 'Association Between Cancer-free
Survival and Telomere DNA Content in Prostate Tumors',
Journal of Urology, 173 (February 2005), p. 610

Karayi, M. K. and A. F. Markham, 'Molecular Biology of
Prostate Cancer', *Prostate Cancer and Prostatic Diseases*, 7 (2004),
pp. 6–20

Rhodes, Daniel R., K. Shanker, Nandan Deshpande, Radhika
Varambally, Debashis Ghosh, Terrence Barrette, Akhilesh
Pandey and Arul M. Chinnaiyan, 'Large-Scale Meta-
Analysis of Cancer Microarray Data Identifies Common
Transcriptional Profiles of Neoplastic Transformation and
Progression', *Proceedings of the National Academy of Sciences*, 101
(June 2004), pp. 9309–14

Salmon, Cynthia, Mark G. Knize, Frances N. Panteleakos,
Rebekah W. Wu, David O. Nelson and James S. Felton,
'Minimization of Heterocyclic Amines and Thermal
Inactivation of Escherichia Coli in Fried Ground Beef',
Journal of the National Cancer Institute, 92 (2000), pp. 1773–8

Tricoli, James, Mason Schoenfeld and Barbara A. Conley,
'Detection of Prostate Cancer and Predicting Progression:
Current and Future Diagnostic Markers', *Clinical Cancer
Research*, 10 (June 2004), pp. 3943–53

Vogelstein, Bert and Kenneth W. Kinzler, 'Cancer Genes and the
    Pathways They Control', *Nature Medicine*, 10 (August 2004),
    pp. 789–99

Epilogue: the future
American Cancer Society, *Breast Cancer Facts and Figures, 2003–
    2004* (2005)
—, *Cancer Facts and Figures, 2005* (2005)
Cancer Research UK, *CancerStats Monograph 2004* (2004)
Dalgleish, Angus, Mike Richards and Karol Sikora, 'Prevention',
    in *Cancer 2025* by Karol Sikora
Donovan, R. J., O. B. Carter, G. Jalleh and S. C. Jones, 'Changes
    in Beliefs about Cancer in Western Australia, 1964–2001',
    Medical Journal of Australia (2004)
Dzik-Jurasz, Andrzej, Malcolm Mason and Harvey Schipper,
    'Imaging', in *Cancer 2025* by Karol Sikora
Ellis, Ian, John Fox and Bill Gullick, 'Diagnosis', in *Cancer 2025* by
    Karol Sikora
Epstein, Samuel, *Cancer-Gate: How to Win the Losing Cancer War*
    (Baywood Publishing, 2005)
Goldberg, Paul and Kirsten Boyd Goldberg, 'Special Report:
    The NCI 2015 Goal', *Cancer Letter*, 14 February 2003
Jones, Alison, 'Reduction in Mortality from Breast Cancer',
    British Medical Journal, 330 (29 January 2005), pp. 205–6
Kunkler, Ian, Nick James and Jane Maher, 'Radiotherapy', in
    Cancer 2025 by Karol Sikora
Lehtinen, Matti and Jorma Paavonen, 'Vaccination Against
    Human Papillomaviruses Shows Great Promise', *The Lancet*,
    364 (13 November 2004), pp. 1731–2
Morrell, Jill and Joanna Pryce, *Work and Cancer: How Cancer Affects
    Working Lives* (CancerBacup, 2005)
O'Brien, Catherine, 'The Silent Killer: How Britain is Leading
    the Fight Against Ovarian Cancer', *The Times*, 17 January
    2005
Schwartz, L. M., S. Woloshin, F. J. Fowler Jr and H. G. Welch,
    'Enthusiasm for Cancer Screening in the United States',
    Journal of the American Medical Association, 291 (7 January 2004),
    pp. 71–8

Sikora, Karol, *Cancer 2025: The Future of Cancer Care* (Expert
    Review of Anticancer Therapies, 2004)
Sikora, Karol and Olivia Sims, 'Cancer 2025: An Introduction',
    in *Cancer 2025* by Karol Sikora

Notes

From Ancient Times: Incipience

6   [*When the first man stood upright*] See Greaves, *Cancer*, pp. 8–10.

6   [*One of the earliest written texts*] See Micozzi, 'Disease in Antiquity', p. 838; also in Spigelman and Bentley, 'Cancer in Ancient Egypt'.

6   [*A thousand years later*] See Greaves, *Cancer*, p. 10.

6   [*By 400 BC*] See more detail in Retsas, *Paleo-Oncology*.

7   [*a tiny proportion of all deaths*] This is discussed in Micozzi, 'Disease in Antiquity'. Ricci *et al.* in 'Some Considerations about the Incidence of Neoplasms in Human History' detail the slow increase in incidence during the millennium after Christ.

7   [*two-thirds of cancer cases*] In Cancer Research UK's *CancerStats*. American Cancer Society's *Cancer Facts and Figures* (p. 3) states that 76 per cent of cancers occur in the over-55s.

7   [*Why these symptoms develop*] From Reedy, 'Galen on Cancer and Related Diseases', p. 229.

7   [*Galen was famous as the doctor*] From chapter 15, 'The Life and Career of Galen', in Nutton, *Ancient Medicine*.

7   [*swellings which are contrary to nature*] From Reedy, 'Galen on Cancer and Related Diseases', p. 229.

8   [*Egyptians were supposedly at particular risk*] See Nutton, 'Managing a Metaphor', p. 6.

8   [*I have done as much*] Cited in Porter, *The Greatest Benefit to Mankind*, p. 77.

10   [*The first roots of this scientific medicine*] See Porter, Ibid., p. 211.

10   [*the family of a Dorset girl*] Cited in Jackson, 'The Strange Case of Ms Elizabeth Trevers'.

11   [*you can seldom find a convent*] Cited in Greaves, *Cancer*, p. 144.

11   [*cancer remained a rare disease of older women*] See Greaves, Ibid., p. 15. Almost ten times as many women as men developed it in Verona.

11   [*old methods were used*] See De Moulin, 'Historical Notes on Breast Cancer', p. 211.

11   [*the surgeon should therefore*] Cited in De Moulin, Ibid., p. 215.

11   [*An ingenious Dutchman*] See De Moulin, Ibid., p. 213.

12   [*the first hospital*] From Porter, *The Greatest Benefit to Mankind*, p. 387; also in Greaves, *Cancer*, p. 15.

12   [*tumours were caused by 'acrimony'*] See De Moulin, 'Historical Notes on Breast Cancer', p. 208.

13   [*De sedibus et causis morborum*] See Porter, *The Greatest Benefit to Mankind*, p. 263.

14   [*thrust up narrow*] Cited in Greaves, *Cancer*, p. 199.

14   [*Nonetheless, tuberculosis*] See Sontag, *Illness as Metaphor.*

15   [*The first statistical analysis*] See Greaves, *Cancer*, p. 15.

15   [*intention being solely that of cooperating*] See Baillie *et al.*, 'The Medical Committee of the Society'.

15   [*shortage of bodies*] Even Rudolf Virchow complained that there were insufficient bodies for his studies in 1939, in *Letters to His Parents*, p. 18.

15   [*Many families refused*] See Richardson, *Death, Dissection and the Destitute*, p. 93.

16   [*a riot in New York*] See Sappol, *A Traffic of Dead Bodies*, p. 108.

1831: Surgery

17   [*On Saturday 9 April 1831*] See *The Lancet*, 'Guy's Hospital'.

17   [*an enormous tumour*] Although contemporary reports describe this as a tumour, I am told by Professor Michael Baum that modern doctors would call it a hydrocele, a collection of fluid in the scrotum which is not cancerous.

17   [*of a nature and extent*] Quoted in *The Lancet*, 'Guy's Hospital'.

18   [*a great number of persons of all ranks*] Ibid.

18   [*annals of surgery*] Ibid.

18   [*Sir Astley Cooper*] See the acerbic biography by Geoffrey Keynes.

18   [*arriving at the royal chamber*] A detail from Fisher, *Joseph Lister*, p. 125.

18   [*The quality which is considered*] Quoted in Cooper, *Lectures*, p. 8.

19   [*firmly set his teeth*] See *The Lancet*, 'Guy's Hospital'.

20   [*I think that*] See Simpson, 'Letter'.

20   [*terror that surpasses*] Quoted in Porter, *The Greatest Benefit to Mankind*, p. 365.

21   [*The callow 27-year-old*] See books by Wolfe, Fradin and Duncum listed in the Bibliography.

22   [*for the strongest influences*] Quoted in Wolfe, *Tarnished Idol*, p. 81.

22   [*At the appointed time*] See Ayer, 'An Eye-witness Account'.

23   [*to my great surprise*] Quoted in Duncum, *The Development of Inhalation Anaesthesia*, p. 110.

23   [*we have conquered pain*] Cited in Fradin, *We Have Conquered Pain*, p. 67.

24   [*Isabella Pim discovered a large lump*] This story is from Cameron, *Reminiscences of Lister*; Fisher, *Joseph Lister*; Godlee, *Lord Lister* and Guthrie, *Lord Lister*.

24   [*rather than infection*] Cited in Fisher, *Joseph Lister*, p. 145.

25   [*of various low forms of life*] See Lister, 'A New Method of Treating Compound Fracture', p. 327.

25   [*No one can say*] and [*I felt his true kindness*] Cited in Godlee, *Lord Lister*, p. 211.

25   [*I suppose before this reaches*] Quoted in Fisher, *Joseph Lister*, p. 148.

26   [*saw how much it cost him*] In Cameron, *Reminiscences of Lister*, p. 32.

26   [*I may say*] Cited in Fisher, *Joseph Lister*, p. 148.

26   [*now he presented*] Ibid., p. 149.

26   [*As there appears*] Lister, 'On the Antiseptic Principle,' p. 246.

27   [*Where are these little beasts*] John Hughes Bennett, quoted in Porter, *The Greatest Benefit to Mankind*, p. 372.

27 [*a 43-year-old woman called Therese Heller*] See Absolon,
Developmental Technology, p. 95.

28 [*how history would judge him*] See Absolon, *The Surgeon's Surgeon*,
p. 7.

28 [*There was not the slightest confusion*] From a letter quoted in full
in Absolon, *Developmental Technology*.

29 [*I was happily*] Ibid., p. 97.

29 [*the tumour recurred*], See Absolon, *The Surgeon's Surgeon*, p. 7.

1845: Cells

31 [*a 50-year-old cook*] See Virchow, 'Weisses Blut'.

31 [*raspberry jelly*] Described in Lesky, *The Vienna Medical School*.

33 [*Rudolf Virchow was the son*] For more, see Introduction to
Virchow, *Letters to His Parents*.

33 [*Those were the days of great*] From Virchow, *Cellular Pathology*,
p. 71, in Rather, *Disease, Life and Man*.

33 [*Virchow began by*] Virchow describes his method in *A
Description and Explanation of the Method of Performing Post-
mortem Examinations*.

34 [*a truly Danaidean task*] From Virchow, *Letters to His Parents*, p.
61.

34 [*Life is, in essence*] In Rather, *A Commentary*, p. 3.

36 [*Virchow made a speech*] See Virchow, *Letters to His Parents*, p. 61.

36 [*new fangled*] Ibid., p. 62; Virchow also writes, 'The old
military physicians were profoundly shocked at the new
wisdom.'

36 [*duller*] Ibid.

36 [*It is the privilege*] Virchow, *Cellular Pathology*, p. 135.

37 [*he was overcome with sadness*] Ibid., p. 139; he says, 'We have
rarely read one with sadder feelings.'

37 [*blends its hypotheses*] Ibid., p. 132.

37 [*natural science into*] Ibid.

37 [*monstrous*] Ibid., p. 136.

37 [*Now a great uproar*] Virchow, *Letters to His Parents*, p. 70.

38 [*scientific marketplace*] in Rather, 'Virchow's Review of
Rokitansky's Handbuch', p. 130.

39 [*advance his career*] Virchow, *Letters to His Parents*, p. 66.

40   [*Archiv für Pathologie*] Virchow talks about the launch in *Letters to his Parents*, p. 71.

40   [*true science possesses*] Virchow, 'Standpoints in Scientific Medicine', p. 29.

40   [*Side by side*] Virchow, *Letters to His Parents*, p. 72.

40   [*I have a keen desire*] Ibid., p. 75.

40   [*the apathy, this animal servility*] Ibid.

40   [*one sees here quite*] Ibid., p. 77.

40   [*into the social sphere*] See Schlumberger, 'Rudolf Virchow', p. 150.

40   [*On the day of his return*] See Virchow, *Letters to his Parents*, pp. 80–81.

41   [*At this moment*] Ibid., p. 82.

41   [*rusty sabre*] In Boyd, *Rudolf Virchow*, p. 26.

41   [*relatively insignificant*] Virchow, *Letters to His Parents*, p. 84.

41   [*The look of Berlin*] Ibid., p. 86.

41   [*I regard it as my civic duty*] See Schlumberger, 'Rudolf Virchow', p.152.

42   [*Virchow avoided dismissal*] Virchow, *Letters to His Parents*, p. 105.

42   [*playground for my hitherto*] Ibid., p. 110.

42   [*Politically all is stagnation*] Cited in Boyd, *Rudolph Virchow*, p. 50.

42   [*We find ourselves*] Ibid., p. 52.

43   [*multiply by continuous*] Quoted in Kisch, 'Forgotten Leaders', p. 260.

43   [[*Remak*] *finally insists*] Ibid.

43   [*when a professorship in pathology*] See Virchow, *Letters to His Parents*, p. 127.

43   [*Virchow was offered*] Ibid., p. 129.

43   [*accused Virchow of plagiarising*] Described in Parker, 'On the Discovery of Leukaemia'.

44   [*I must be excused*] Quoted in Rather, *A Commentary*, p. 63.

44   [*form a free state*] Cited in Ackerknecht, *Rudolf Virchow*, p. 83.

47   [*Under such circumstances*] Darwin, *The Origin of Species* (1859; repub. Signet Classics), p. 97.

1895: Radiation

50 [*On 8 November 1895*] See Porter, *The Greatest Benefit to Mankind*, p. 605.

51 [*The phenomenon itself*] Quoted in the *New York Times*, 4 February 1896.

51 [*With the discovery of germs*] See Porter, *The Greatest Benefit to Mankind*, p. 427.

52 [*the eighth leading cause*] See Patterson, *The Dread Disease*, p. 32.

52 [*scarlet fever*] Ibid., p. 33.

52 [*Cancer the Crab*] Ibid., p. 31.

52 [*harnessing them against skin and breast cancer*] In Eisenberg, *Radiology*, p. 485.

53 [*a 16-year-old girl*] Described by Béclère, 'Le traitement médical'.

56 [*Curie's scientific career*] See Porter, *The Greatest Benefit to Mankind*, p. 607.

56 [*cataclysm of atomic*] Cited in Curie, *Marie Curie*, p. 192.

57 [*Aladdin's Lamp*] From the *Medical Record: A Weekly Journal of Medicine and Surgery*, 17 October 1903.

57 [*one of the most terrible scourges*] Cited in Quinn, *Marie Curie*, p. 389.

57 [*I feel myself invaded*] Cited in Reid, *Marie Curie*, p. 134.

57 [*scientific matters*] Ibid., p. 246

58 [*What it means*] Ibid., p. 249.

58 [*I saw a pale*] In Meloney's Introduction to Marie Curie's *Pierre Curie*, p. 5.

58 [*Thomas Edison's well-equipped laboratory*] Ibid., p. 4.

58 [*had contributed to the progress*] Ibid., p. 6.

58 [*To this end*] See Reid, *Marie Curie*, p. 251.

58 [*1921 edition of The Delineator*] Cited in Quinn, *Marie Curie*, p. 387.

59 [*her salary was also supplemented*] Ibid., p. 387.

59 [*Grain insufficient*] Cited in Reid, *Marie Curie*, p. 252.

59 [*The gram of radium*] Ibid., p. 254.

59 [*the marching bands*] Described in Curie, *Marie Curie*, p. 339.

60 [*American doctors were more cautious*] See Clarke, *Radium Girls*, p. 59.

61 [*Nevertheless there can be*] Quoted in the *New York Times*, 12 May 1921.

61   [*Meloney sent for a tailor*] See Curie, *Marie Curie*, p. 319.

61   [*Shy, weary and disinterested*] Cited in Reid, *Marie Curie*, p. 263.

61   [*Symbol and Volume*] In Quinn, *Marie Curie*, p. 397.

61   [*This little phial*] Ibid.

61   [*my work with radium*] Ibid., p. 398.

62   [*There is no case*] Ibid.

63   [*Claudius Regaud*] See del Regato, *Radiological Oncologists*.

65   [*a most terrible*] Cited in Clark, *Radium Girls*, p. 35.

65   [*The afflicted convened*] Ibid.

65   [*work in our application*] Ibid., p. 38.

66   [*This first court case*] Ibid., p. 115.

66   [*a horrible jaw problem*] Ibid.

66   [*Perhaps radium has*] Cited in Quinn, *Marie Curie*, p. 416.

66   [*She will be*] Ibid., p. 415.

67   [*Grace Fryer*] See Clark, *Radium Girls*, p. 120.

67   [*If radium has unknown*] Quoted in Kovarik, 'Radium Girls'.

67   [*Five women smile*] Ibid.

67   [*damnable travesty of*] Ibid.

68   [*settlement of $15,000*] Clark, *Radium Girls*, p. 135.

1930: Causes

70   [*A grim spectre*] Carson, *Silent Spring*, p. 22.

70   [*A Fable for Tomorrow*] Ibid., p. 21.

70   [*Everywhere was a shadow of death*] Ibid.

71   [*For the first time in the history*] Ibid., p. 31.

71   [*With the dawn of the industrial era*] Ibid., p. 193.

71   [*have entered the environment*] Ibid., pp. 193, 195.

72   [*foremost authority*] Ibid., p. 195.

72   [*Wilhelm Hueper*] Hueper's life story is drawn mostly from his own memoirs, *Adventures of a Physician in Occupational Cancer*; there is also a biography in Robert Proctor, *Cancer Wars*, p. 37.

72   [*a monster that is more insatiable*] Quoted in Patterson, *The Dread Disease*, p. 82.

73   [*a series of competing ideas*] See Proctor, *Cancer Wars*, p. 32.

73   [*viruses*] Ibid., p. 105.

73   [*Even Freudian psychoanalysts*] Wilhelm Reich would eventually write *The Cancer Biopathy* in 1948 as the definitive statement

on the subject, although the idea had existed for years before.

73   [*Nobody knows what*] 'Miss Gee', in Auden, *Collected Poems*, p. 55.

75   [*distinctly alarmed*] Hueper, *Adventures of a Physician*, p. 140.

75   [*a new industrial hazard*] Ibid.; also in Proctor, *Cancer Wars*, p. 38.

75   [*studied for their toxic*] Hueper, *Adventures of a Physician*, pp. 140, 142.

75   [*impairing the availability*] Ibid.

75   [*We decided to test our luck*] Ibid., p. 143; for a longer discussion, see Proctor, *The Nazi War on Cancer*, p. 35.

75   [*Heil Hitler*] Quoted Ibid., p. 13.

76   [*the simpler and more natural*] Cited Ibid., p. 24.

76   [*cancer prevention*] Cited Ibid., pp. 24, 25.

76   [*Hueper's first job interview*] See Hueper, *Adventures of a Physician*, p. 144.

76   [*new race of cells*] Quoted in Proctor, *Nazi War on Cancer*, p. 47.

77   [*The adventure was over*] Hueper, *Adventures of a Physician*, p. 145.

78   [*rise in the modern*] Hueper, *Occupational Tumors and Allied Diseases*, p. 4.

78   [*dyes, mordants, explosives*] Ibid., p. 40.

79   [*communistic tendencies*] See Hueper, *Adventures of a Physician*, chapter 4.

81   [*At the age of 36*] From Doll, 'The First Reports on Smoking and Lung Cancer', and an interview with Richard Doll.

81   [*increased sixfold*] From Doll, 'Smoking and Carcinoma of the Lung'.

82   [*If I had to put money*] Quoted in Le Fanu, *The Rise and Fall of Modern Medicine*, p. 49.

82   [*Franz Müller*] There is a longer discussion about this in Proctor, *Nazi War on Cancer*, pp. 194–6.

82   [*extremely heavy smokers*] Ibid., p. 196.

83   [*Best of luck*] Ibid., p. 209.

83   [*In London in*] The following is taken from Doll and Hill, 'Smoking and Lung Cancer'.

84   [*50 times as*] From Ibid., p. 747.

85   [*entirely new method*] See Doll, *Cohort Studies*.

86   [*batches of Lucky Strike*] from Kluger, *Ashes to Ashes*, p. 160.

86   [*suspected human carcinogen*] Ibid., p. 162.

86   [*Doll and Hill followed*] From Doll and Hill, 'The Mortality of Doctors in Relation to Their Smoking Habits'.

87   [*no convincing clinical*] Kluger, *Ashes to Ashes*, p. 169.

88   [*The acceptance of the cigarette theory*] Hueper, *Adventures of a Physician*, p. 183.

88   [*He was German*] Interview with Richard Doll.

88   [*In 1956, Doll and Hill*] Cited in Kluger, *Ashes to Ashes*, p. 195.

89   [*I then realized*] Carson, *Silent Spring*, p. 9.

89   [*a sincere, unusually well-informed*] See Brooks, *House of Life*, p. 255.

90   [*suspicious enough to*] Leopold, *A Darker Ribbon*, p. 127.

90   [*curious, hard swelling*] Ibid., p. 129.

90   [*Among the most eminent*] Carson, *Silent Spring*, p. 213.

91   [*Cigarette smoking is associated*] From Advisory Committee to the Surgeon General, *Smoking and Health*, p. 31.

93   [*Man has put the vast majority of carcinogens*] Carson, *Silent Spring*, p. 213.

94   [*the natural world is full of chemicals*] There is a wider discussion of this idea in Proctor, *Cancer Wars*, p. 134.

94   [*the second major cause of cancer is diet*] It should be noted that this theory is disputed by Le Fanu, *The Rise and Fall of Modern Medicine*, p. 354.

94   [*one experiment showed that a burger*] Salmon *et al.*, 'Minimization of Heterocyclic Amines'.

95   [*our behaviour as a species is so different*] For a longer discussion of this, see Greaves, *Cancer*.

1947: Chemotherapy

98   [*the 4-year-old girl*] This story is largely drawn from Farber *et al.*, 'Temporary Remissions in Acute Leukemia in Children'.

99   [*According to one of her doctors*] From Pochedly, 'Dr James A. Wolff II First Successful Chemotherapy of Acute Leukemia'.

99   [*In the minds of most physicians*] From Alfred Gilman, 'The Initial Clinical Trial of Nitrogen Mustard', p. 557.

100 [*The atmosphere of the Children's Hospital*] From Fergusson, 'A Living Legend of Pediatric Oncology Nursing', pp. 229–38.

101 [*A change of this magnitude*] Farber *et al.*, 'Temporary Remissions in Acute Leukemia in Children', p. 787.

101 [*well developed and nourished*] Ibid., p. 788.

102 [*doctors conducted warfare*] From Pochedly, 'Dr James A. Wolff II First Successful Chemotherapy of Acute Leukemia', p. 452.

102 [*but eventually Janeway*] See Mercer, 'The Team'.

104 [*a 2-year-old boy*] This is Case 5 from Farber *et al.*, 'Temporary Remissions in Acute Leukemia in Children'.

104 [*two-and-a-half-year-old girl*] Case 4 from Ibid.

105 [*Farber rebuked Mercer*] See Pochedly, 'Dr James A. Wolff II First Successful Chemotherapy of Acute Leukemia', p. 452.

105 [*in excellent physical condition*] Farber *et al.*, 'Temporary Remissions in Acute Leukemia in Children', p. 788.

105 [*gone round the bend*] 'Dr James A. Wolff II First Successful Chemotherapy of Acute Leukemia', p. 453.

106 [*The child is Linda Dias*] *New York Times*, 16 April 1947.

106 [*Very rapid progress*] Cited in Patterson, *The Dread Disease*, p. 142.

106 [*scourge that kills more*] Ibid., p. 152.

108 [*If the entire atmosphere*] From Farber *et al.*, 'Advances in Chemotherapy of Cancer in Man', p. 6.

108 [*never allowed us*] Galbraith, *A Life in Our Times*, p. 278.

109 [*I think it is sad indeed*] US Congress, 'Department of Labor and Federal Security Agency Appropriations for 1953'; Hearings, 82nd Congress, 2nd Session, 20 February 1952, p. 197.

109 [*Rhoads had employed*] See Lasker, 'The Unforgettable Character of Dusty Rhoads'.

110 [*this very, very skinny*] From 'The Reminiscences of Mary Lasker', in the Oral History Collection, Columbia University, 18 April 1966.

111 [*This little fellow*] Quoted in Rettig, *Cancer Crusade*, p. 57.

111 [*Inevitably as I see it*] Quoted in Patterson, *The Dread Disease*, p. 196.

112 [*By 1957, chemotherapy drug testing*] See Goodman and Walsh, *The Story of Taxol.*

112 [*The mass and mechanized*] Gellhorn, 'Invited Remarks on the Current State of Research', p. 6.

112 [*Still his burning ambition*] Lasker, 'The Unforgettable Character of Dusty Rhoads'.

115 [*Howard Earle Skipper*] See Le Fanu, *The Rise and Fall of Modern Medicine*, pp. 138–55; also in Ibid.

115 [*We began wondering*] In Laszlo, *The Cure of Childhood Leukemia*, p. 234.

116 [*James Eversull*] See his story in Ibid., p. 244.

116 [*We had to convert*] Ibid., p. 234.

116 [*I remember the other children*] Ibid., p. 244.

1969: The War on Cancer

118 [*Mary Lasker boarded*] From Mary Lasker's office diary of 1969. Much of this chapter is drawn from papers in her archive at Columbia University as well as from Richard Rettig's magisterial *Cancer Crusade.*

118 [*$181 million*] From Rettig, *Cancer Crusade*, p. 30.

119 [*the same talents for organization*] From a memorandum, 'Need for a Senate Commission on the Conquest of Cancer as a National Goal by 1976', 9 January 1970, in 'The Reminiscences of Mary Lasker', the Oral History Research Office, Collection of Columbia University.

119 [*Lasker had little patience*] Throughout Lasker's annual Oral History interviews she disdains basic research. At the same time, she steadfastly gave the Lasker Award for Basic Medical Research.

119 [*perverse … to the patient*] from 'The Reminiscences of Mary Lasker', 7 January 1972.

119 [*Lasker reached the office*] See Rettig, *Cancer Crusade*, p. 80.

119 [*$650 million*] See Garb, *Cure for Cancer*, p. 298.

119 [*with the least possible delay*] Ibid., p. v.

120 [*George Bush*] In actual fact Yarborough failed to win the primary and left the Senate; see Rettig, *Cancer Crusade*, p. 87.

120 [*very, very disorganized*] See Ibid., p. 81.

121 [*Lasker then paid $22,000*] Ibid., pp. 79–81.

122 [*A piece of bad news*] See P. B. Medawar and J. S. Medawar, *Aristotle to Zoos: A Philosophical Dictionary of Biology* (Oxford University Press, 1985), p. 32.

122 [*the discovery in 1964*] See M. A. Epstein, B. G. Achong and Y. M. Barry, 'Virus Particles in Cultured Lymphoblasts from Burkitt's Lymphoma', *The Lancet*, 28 March 1964, pp. 702–3.

123 [*Special Virus Cancer Program*] For a broader discussion of the SVCP, see Weinberg, *Racing to the Beginning of the Road*, pp. 66–83.

123 [*Building 41*] See Auerbach, 'Institute to Probe Causes of Cancer'.

123 [*a survey of patients*] 'Tests Link Some Cancers to Virus', in *Washington Post*, 5 December 1969.

124 [*developed a new hypothesis*] Huebner and Todaro, 'Oncogenes of RNA Tumor Viruses'.

124 [*The Senate soon passed*] See Rettig, *Cancer Crusade*, p. 81.

125 [*Scientists have found*] Auerbach, 'New Virus "Strongly Linked" to Breast Cancer'.

125 [*Yarborough asked Lasker*] From 'The Reminiscences of Mary Lasker', 29 December 1970.

125 [*Her choice was Benno Schmidt*], Actually Schmidt was suggested by Laurence Rockefeller.

125 [*Throughout that autumn*] See Rettig, *Cancer Crusade*, p. 102.

126 [*While Republican members*] Ibid., p. 122.

126 [*As Kennedy might be … to achieve this goal*] Ibid., p. 125.

128 [*uncritical zealots*] Ibid., p. 133.

129 [*it will not speed*] Ibid., p. 235.

129 [*The 325,000 patients*] Ibid., p. 217.

129 [*For this legislation*] Ibid., p. 278.

129 [*It was a beautiful day*] From 'The Reminiscences of Mary Lasker', 7 January 1972, p. 742.

130 [*People at the National Institutes of Health*] Ibid., 8 July 1978, p. 748.

130 [*A government study*] See Culliton, 'Cancer: Select Committee Calls Virus Program Closed Shop'.

130 [*There did not*] Ibid., p. 1111.

132 [*Thank you for*] from Mary Lasker archive, Kennedy file.

133 [*You have made*] Quoted in Lerner, *The Breast Cancer Wars*, p. 173.

133 [*Mary Lasker wanted*] Interview with Mathilde Krim.

133 [*Only one place in the world*] In Hall, *A Commotion in the Blood*, p. 160.

133 [*simply thrilling*] Lasker, 'History of Interferon', p. 20-296.

133 [*I am perfectly aware*] Ibid., p. 20-795.

134 [*Now of course*] Ibid., p. 20-797

135 [*utter bliss*] Quoted in Hall, *Commotion in the Blood*, p. 201.

135 [*the date on which*] Wade, 'Cloning Gold Rush Turns Basic Biology into Big Business'.

135 [*We paid heavily*] Jordan Gutterman, quoted in Panem, *The Interferon Crusade*, p. 23.

136 [*Researchers found themselves*] see Panen, *The Interferon Crusade*, pp. 75–8.

136 [*They did not offer*] Quoted in Hall, *A Commotion in the Blood*, p. 208.

137 [*mortality rates have shown … war on cancer*] Bailar and Smith, 'Progress Against Cancer?'.

137 [*I think that our efforts*] 'The Reminiscences of Mary Lasker', 10 August 1981, p. 219.

138 [*I don't understand this*] Ibid.

1979: **Alternatives**

140 [*a large, painful lump*] See Brohn, *Gentle Giants*, p. 4; the story is also drawn from Brohn's interview in *The Gentle Way With Cancer?*, a six-part documentary series, broadcast on BBC2, March 1983.

140 [*his management of my crisis*] Brohn, *Gentle Giants*, p. 2.

141 [*if the hospital*] Ibid., p. 7.

141 [*a big bundle*] Ibid., p. 6.

142 [*a pathogen alongside resistant strains*] Ibid., p. 39.

142 [*Other critics*] See Moss, *The Cancer Industry*.

143 [*The most significant feeling I had*] Brohn, *Gentle Giants*, p. 4.

144 [*I knew that my cancer*] Ibid.

144 [*this was our first tentative offering … that night*] Ibid., p. 18.

145 [*I mastered them*] Ibid., p. 24.

145 [*may turn out to be*] Quoted in Hager, *Force of Nature*, p. 598.

146 [*It's a bugger*] Brohn, *Gentle Giants*, p. 35.

148 [*But they arrive at this ordinary house*] From *A Gentle Way With Cancer?*

148 [*Inspire yourself with the thought*] Brohn, 'Working Your Way Back to Health', Bristol Cancer Help Centre pamphlet, March 1982.

149 [*it is a fact that people*] Alec Forbes, 'Cancer and Its Non-toxic Treatment', Bristol Cancer Help Centre pamphlet.

149 [*The people who come here*] From *A Gentle Way with Cancer?*

150 [*Carl asked him to picture*] Simonton, Matthews-Simonton and James Creighton, *Getting Well Again*, p. 7.

151 [*Do the therapies work?*] Forbes, 'Cancer and Its Non-toxic treatment'.

151 [*Penny Brohn promoted the drug*] See Brohn, *The Bristol Programme*, p. 74.

152 [*at physical, emotional*] Quoted in *The Times*, 'Healing Backed by Prince'.

152 [*in cancer as in most*] *The Times* editorial, 10 August 1983.

154 [*Sir Walter Bodmer*] See Bagenal *et al.*, 'Survival of Patients with Breast Cancer Attending Bristol Cancer Help Centre'.

154 [*I have seen no evidence*] In *The Gentle Way with Cancer?*

154 [*I think ... thing that is important*] Ibid.

155 [*This means that in a few years' time*] Brohn, *The Bristol Programme*, p. 6.

155 [*She was struggling ... get it right*] Interview with Michael Wetzler.

156 [*bald, sleek, fat*] Appleyard, 'Chaos Creeps up on Science as Two Medicines Collide'.

156 [*These results show*] Bagenal *et al.*, 'Survival of Patients with Breast Cancer Attending Bristol Cancer Help Centre', p. 609.

156 [*there might be some element*] Sherman, 'Cancer Patients at Holistic Centre'.

157 [*The following day*] See Walker, *Dirty Medicine*, p. 585.

157 [*McElwain rolled his eyes*] Appleyard, 'Chaos Creeps up on Science as Two Medicines Collide'.

157 [*impossible to imagine*] Ibid.

157 [*possible weakness*] Hayes and Carpenter, 'Bristol Cancer Help Centre'.

157 [*We regret that our paper*] Chilvers, McElwain *et al.*, Letter, *The Lancet*, 10 November 1990.

158 [*throughout the 1980s the public mood*] See Eisenberg *et al.*, 'Unconventional Medicine in the United States'; see also Downer *et al.*, 'Pursuit and Practice of Complementary Therapies': 16 per cent of cancer patients are taking unconventional medicine.

159 [*The Bristol Cancer Help Centre*] See Cooke, *The Bristol Approach to Living With Cancer*.

160 [*My fight against cancer*] From Ausubel, *When Healing Becomes a Crime*, p. 17.

1982: Genes

164 [*Robert Weinberg*] The narrative from this story is drawn largely from Weinberg, *Racing to the Beginning of the Road*, and Angier, *Natural Obsessions*, as well as interviews conducted by the author with Robert Weinberg, Chaiho Shih and Michael Wigler.

164 [*We had relatively … Mother Nature*] Weinberg, *Racing to the Beginning of the Road*, p. 6.

166 [*it was an epiphany*] Ibid., p. 137.

166 [*skin of my arse*] Interview with Weinberg.

166 [*But Goldfarb told Weinberg*] See Angier, *Natural Obsessions*, p. 75.

167 [*I was reluctant*] Ibid., p. 76.

168 [*what kind of crazy*] Ibid.

168 [*After twenty-five attempts*] Weinberg, *Racing to the Beginning of the Road*, p. 148.

168 [*In April 1978*] Ibid., p. 137.

168 [*My depression deepened*] Ibid., p. 142.

170 [*When Shih arrived*] Quoted in Angier, *Natural Obsessions*, p. 91.

170 [*He suggested that they procure*] Ibid., p. 93.

171 [*My talk evoked*] Weinberg, *Racing to the Beginning of the Road*, p. 152; Shih *et al.*, 'Passage of Phenotypes of Chemically Transformed Cells'.

171 [*not very convincing demonstration*] Weinberg, *Racing to the Beginning of the Road*, p. 153.

171 [*that was a turning point*] Quoted in Angier, *Natural Obsessions*, p. 98.

171 [*People made fun of Bob*], Mariano Barbacid, quoted Ibid., p. 96.

172 [*Shih and Weinberg submitted a paper*] Shih *et al.*, 'Tranforming Genes of Carcinomas and Neuroblastomas Introduced into Mouse Fibroblasts'.

173 [*I was tired … to be fools*] Weinberg, *Racing to the Beginning of the Road*, p. 166.

174 [*We needed to move in close*] Ibid., p. 166.

174 [*They were laughing at Bob*] Quoted in Angier, *Natural Obsessions*, p. 109.

174 [*We were driven to this race*] Interview with Weinberg.

175 [*I was depressed*] Interview with Chiaho Shih.

175 [*It was incredibly exciting*] Interview with Michael Wigler.

175 [*We were beaten*] Weinberg, *Racing to the Beginning of the Road*, p. 175.

175 [*All three groups published*] Shih and Weinberg, 'Isolation of a Transforming Sequence'; Barbacid *et al.*, 'Oncogenes in Human Tumor Cell Lines'; Goldfarb *et al.*, 'Isolation and Preliminary Characterization of a Human Transforming Gene'.

175 [*we have provided direct proof*] Shih and Weinberg, 'Isolation of a Transforming Sequence'.

176 [*The excitement surrounding*] Weinberg, 'Oncogenes of Human Tumor Cells'.

177 [*Tabin's first action*] See Angier, *Natural Obsessions*, p. 121.

178 [*I was getting desperate*] Weinberg, *Racing to the Beginning of the Road*, p. 195.

179 [*It is one of the most startling*] *Nature*, 'Anatomy of a Cancer Gene', p. 103.

179 [*Human cancer research is now moving*] *New York Times*, 24 October 1982.

179 [*According to some historians*] See Fujimora, *Crafting Science*, Morange, 'From the Regulatory Vision of Cancer to the Oncogene Paradigm'.

181 [*My first reaction*] Quoted in Angier, *Natural Obsessions*, p. 115.
181 [*was one of those rare*] Weinberg, *Racing to the Beginning of the Road*, p. 182.
181 [*there existed just a few genes*] See Weinberg, 'Fewer and Fewer Oncogenes'.

1992: Prevention
185 [*It has been estimated*] From the National Institute of Health, 'Cancer Facts: Genetic Testing for BRCA1 and BRCA2: It's Your Choice', http://cis.nci.nih.gov/fact/3_62.htm.
186 [*results which he published in his landmark paper*] Fisher *et al.*, 'Five-year Results of a Randomized Clinical Trial Comparing Total Mastectomy and Segmental Mastectomy with or without Radiation in the Treatment of Breast Cancer', *New England Journal of Medicine*, 14 March 1985, pp. 665–73.
187 [*Show me a hero*] Interview with Bernard Fisher.
187 [*Bernard Fisher's Breast Cancer Prevention Trial was launched*] From Fisher *et al.*, 'Tamoxifen for Prevention of Breast Cancer'.
187 [*Samuel Broder had declared it a priority*] Interview with Broder.
187 [*and had allocated $68 million*] Roan, 'Cancer Prevention Trials Open New Era in Medicine'.
187 [*Bernard Fisher and other international researchers*] See Jordan, *Tamoxifen*. Actually the risk reduction for tamoxifen is only for women who have so-called Oestrogen Receptor Positive. About two-thirds of all patients with breast cancer surgery fit into this category.
188 [*Fisher believed that the 175,000*] From Fisher, 'The Evolution of Paradigms for the Management of Breast Cancer', p. 2371.
188 [*drastic, paradigmatic change*] Ibid., p. 2380.
188 [*The risk/benefit ratio*] Fugh-Berman, 'Tamoxifen in Healthy Women'.
188 [*The acceptable risks*] Ibid.
189 [*They are on the frontier*] Interview with Fugh-Berman.
190 [*It was a terrible, frightening thing*] Friedman, 'The Women Who Volunteer for a Cancer-Prevention Study'.
190 [*I think nothing would have dissuaded*] Interview with Renee Rauch.

190 [*Since I've been on the program*] Friedman, 'The Women Who Volunteer for a Cancer-Prevention Study'.

191 [*After attending a meeting … only generally*] Human Resources and Intergovernmental Relations Subcommittee of the Committee on Government Operations, 'Breast Cancer Prevention Study'.

191 [*The most startling discovery*] Ibid., p. 260.

192 [*some of the archaic taboos were being challenged*] See Lerner, *Breast Cancer Wars*, p. 271.

192 [*I still do not appreciate*] Fisher, 'Thoughts From a Journey', p. 2305.

192 [*Of those, twenty-three*] Fisher *et al.*, 'Endometrial Cancer in Tamoxifen-Treated Breast Cancer Patients'.

192 [*deaths from uterine cancers*] Quoted in Seachrist, 'Restating the Risks of Tamoxifen', p. 911.

193 [*though we certainly wouldn't refuse*] Ibid.

193 [*We have conducted a risk-benefit analysis*] Ibid.

195 [*If breast cancer patients*] *New York Times*, 'The Breast Cancer Fabrications'.

196 [*this episode is yet another*] Quoted in Altman, 'Federal Officials to Review Documents'.

196 [*These criticisms have been going on*] Quoted in 'Cancel Tamoxifen Trial, Critics Urge', *San Francisco Chronicle*, 16 March 1994.

196 [*We did that to make sure*] Interview with Samuel Broder.

197 [*My anger and outrage*] House of Representatives, 'Scientific Misconduct in Breast Cancer Research'.

197 [*originally a bad idea*] Ibid.

198 [*The US National Cancer Institute convened a meeting*] The Consensus Report can be found at http://consensus.nih.gov/1997/1997BreastCancerScreening103html.htm.

199 [*the data currently available*] Ibid.

199 [*Each woman should decide*] Ibid.

200 [*Richard Klausner … shocked*] Quoted in Welch, *Should I Be Tested for Cancer?*, p. 127.

200 [*tantamount to a death sentence*] Quoted in Lerner, *Breast Cancer Wars*, p. 244.

200 [*the US Senate unanimously passed*] Wells, 'Mammography and the Politics of Randomised Controlled Trials'.

200 [*private and personal feelings*] *New England Journal of Medicine*, 'Contentious Screening Decisions', 24 April 1997.

201 [*Perhaps … my passionate attention*] Ibid., p. 172.

201 [*The report's most damning comment*] ORI Investigation Report, ORI 94-08, Office of Research Integrity, 28 February 1997.

201 [*the whole Kafqaesque episode*] Quoted in Peto *et al.*, 'The Trials of Dr. Bernard Fisher'.

202 [*This is an extremely emotional*] Transcript of press conference, 6 April 1998.

204 [*biopsies on young male patients*] See Sakr *et al.*, 'The Frequency of Carcinoma and Intraepithelial Neoplasia of the Prostate'.

1999: Targeting Genes

This basis of this chapter has been interviews with Bud Romine, Dr Brian Druker, Alex Matter, Nick Lydon, Suzan McNamara, and Olivia Stone from Novartis's public relations department. Unless otherwise stated, the quotations in this chapter come from my own reporting.

211 [*a chemist called Jürg Zimmerman*] See Vasella, *Magic Cancer Bullet*, p. 48.

211 [*If it's working here*] Quoted in Hardy, 'Drug May Offer Hope to Adults with Leukemia'.

211 [*The Oregonian*] Koglin, 'New Drug May Fight Common Leukemia'.

216 [*Her tragic illness*] Vasella, *Magic Cancer Bullet*, p. 32.

224 [*I felt the risks were high*] Ibid., p. 93.

225 [*We therefore ask for your assurance*] Ibid., p. 116.

226 [*I did not want huge numbers*] Ibid., p. 96.

226 [*Novartis has devoted substantial*] Ibid., p. 118.

2003: The Clocks of Mortality

233 [*Yet it is possible to construct a plausible account*] This account of what happened to Dad is, of course, a fiction. I can never know what happened. Indeed, there remains much scientific debate about which genes are active in prostate cancer, and in what order. However, it is a reasonable construction of

what might have happened. In this, I was helped by Chris Parker at the Institute of Cancer Research, and by the following papers: Rhodes *et al.*, 'Large-Scale Meta-Analysis'; Karayi and Markham, 'Molecular Biology of Prostate Cancer'; Tricoli *et al.*, 'Detection of Prostate Cancer and Predicting Progression'; and Weinberg, *One Renegade Cell.*

Epilogue: The future

244 [*times of survival have been improving*] American Cancer Society, *Cancer Facts and Figures*; Cancer Research UK, *CancerStats Monograph 2004.*

245 [*as well as screening women over 50*] Jones, 'Reduction in Mortality from Breast Cancer'.

246 [*eliminate suffering and death*] Goldberg and Goldberg, 'Special Report: The NCI 2015 Goal'.

246 [*It is like putting a man on the moon*] Ibid., p. 2.

246 [*cancer is an essentially*] Epstein, *Cancer-Gate*, p. 20.

247 [*will be considered a chronic disease*] Sikora and Sims, 'Cancer 2025: An Introduction'.

247 [*Already testing for the protein CA125*] See O'Brien, 'The Silent Killer'.

248 [*to measure the leakiness*] See Dzik-Jurasz *et al.*, 'Imaging', p. 31.

248 [*a new vaccine that guards against*] Lehtinen and Paavonen, 'Vaccination Against Human Papillomaviruses Shows Great Promise'.

249 [*14 million cancer patients*] In Sikora and Sims, 'Cancer 2025: An Introduction'.

250 [*isolation, loss of self-esteem*] Morrell and Pryce, *Work and Cancer.*

250 [*How to Behave with the Ill*] With the permission of Julia Darling's family. The poem is published in *The Poetry Cure*, ed. Julia Darling and Cynthia Fuller (Newcastle University/Bloodaxe, 2005).

Index